IMPULSE

Sex is everywhere in modern society, yet it remains taboo. We all have questions about sex that are too uncomfortable to ask – how do we get reliable answers? In this go-to guide, Drs. Grant and Chamberlain use their clinical expertise to answer the questions you wish you could ask about sex. Questions like: Is my sex drive or sex behavior normal? Can someone have too much sex? Or too little? How has Internet dating and pornography changed sex?

This go-to guide will help you understand common sexual issues, know when to worry (or not) about different sexual behaviors, and learn how our sex lives adapt to changing technology or in times of crisis. It also provides step-by-step advice for dealing with a range of sexual issues, and practical strategies for strengthening relationships.

JON E. GRANT is a Professor of Psychiatry and Behavioral Neuroscience at the University of Chicago where he directs a clinic and research laboratory on addictive, compulsive, and impulsive disorders.

SAMUEL R. CHAMBERLAIN is a Professor of Psychiatry at the University of Southampton. His research and clinical work focus on the neurobiology and treatment of behaviourally addictive disorders – including compulsive sexual behavior problems.

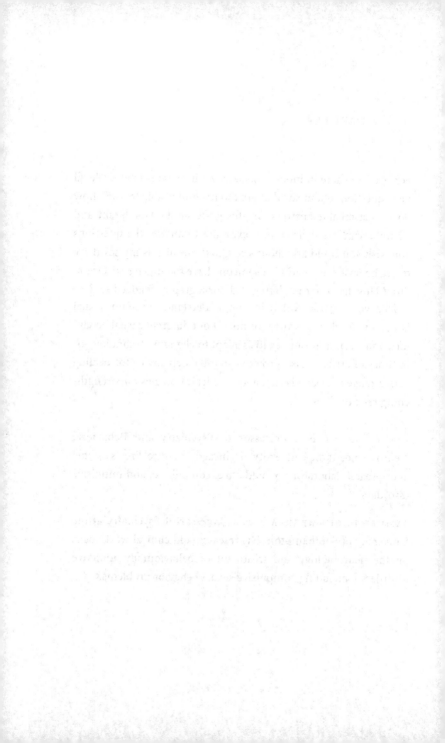

IMPULSE

THE SCIENCE OF SEX AND DESIRE

JON E. GRANT
SAMUEL R. CHAMBERLAIN

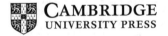

CAMBRIDGE
UNIVERSITY PRESS

University Printing House, Cambridge CB2 8BS, United Kingdom

One Liberty Plaza, 20th Floor, New York, NY 10006, USA

477 Williamstown Road, Port Melbourne, VIC 3207, Australia

314–321, 3rd Floor, Plot 3, Splendor Forum, Jasola District Centre,
New Delhi – 110025, India

103 Penang Road, #05–06/07, Visioncrest Commercial, Singapore 238467

Cambridge University Press is part of the University of Cambridge.

It furthers the University's mission by disseminating knowledge in the pursuit of
education, learning, and research at the highest international levels of excellence.

www.cambridge.org
Information on this title: www.cambridge.org/9781009107976
DOI: 10.1017/9781009106139

First published 2023

Printed in the United Kingdom by TJ Books Limited, Padstow, Cornwall

A catalogue record for this publication is available from the British Library.

Library of Congress Cataloging-in-Publication Data
Names: Grant, Jon E., author. | Chamberlain, Samuel, author.
Title: Sex and desire : the science behind our impulses / Jon E. Grant, University of Chicago,
Samuel R. Chamberlain, University of Cambridge.
Description: First edition. | Cambridge, United Kingdom ; New York, NY : Cambridge
University Press, 2023. | Includes bibliographical references and index.
Identifiers: LCCN 2022012251 (print) | LCCN 2022012252 (ebook) | ISBN 9781009107976
(paperback) | ISBN 9781009106139 (ebook)
Subjects: LCSH: Sex (Psychology) | Sex – Social aspects. | Desire.
Classification: LCC BF692 .G677 2023 (print) | LCC BF692 (ebook) | DDC 155.3–dc23/eng/
20220503
LC record available at https://lccn.loc.gov/2022012251
LC ebook record available at https://lccn.loc.gov/2022012252

ISBN 978-1-009-10797-6 Paperback

CONTENTS

CONTENTS

1   Introduction

For most of us, sex is important. Some of our first close friendships are initiated when we discuss sex – adolescent boys and girls navigating puberty and sexual desires. We may spend countless hours fantasizing about and planning our first sexual experience. Dating for many becomes an important rite of passage. As adults, we look for partners who can provide a satisfying sexual experience. In fact, most people have their first sexual experience long before they fall in love or meet a long-term partner. Sex means different things to different people, and within the same person, sex means different things to us at different times in our lives and changes based on emotional development and life stages. Simply put, sex is complicated.

Even in nonphysical ways, sex seems to permeate our everyday lives. Movies and television series are more enticing if there is a sexual theme. Jokes and conversations are riddled with double entendres. Magazine covers, news, and advertisements sell themselves or products using half-naked people by alluding to fantasies of sex or in many cases graphically telling us about people's sex lives. Sex is obviously more than just a physical act. It also incorporates psychological, social, political, and even spiritual dimensions.

Why is sex so important? The University of Michigan conducted a national poll on healthy aging and found that most older adults (76 percent) reported that sex is an important part of a romantic relationship at any age. The Center for Sexual Health Promotion at the Indiana University School of Public Health has been conducting surveys on sexual health for years, and they recently found that among adolescents, approximately 81 percent described their sexual behavior as anywhere from moderately to extremely pleasurable. Across the lifespan, it appears that for many, sex can be characterized as rewarding. "Rewarding" can mean many things and sex delivers most of them (although sexual reward can be very different for each person). Sex gets our hearts racing; we feel joy, exhilaration, calm, and/or peace. It allows us to escape problems and forget about bills, relatives, and issues at work. For a few minutes or hours, we can feel transported; we feel needed, loved, wanted, and desired. Sex allows us to bond with another person. It is a great mix of reality (the physical nature of sex) melded with the fantasy lives of most of us (we can believe we are sexy even if pudgy and out of shape; we believe our partner is amazing even if we know little about them). This is all very rewarding, and this type of reward is more potent and potentially more reinforcing than most other types of behavior. And so sex is one of the most rewarding behaviors we can engage in, and that reward then leads us to want more sex.

The topic of sex also raises issues regarding the complex interplay between the physical and the mental worlds. Part of sex is obviously physical. Our bodies get stimulated and we respond wanting greater stimulation and ultimately release. The other part of sex, however, exists in our mental universe or space. Beginning in adolescence,

2

sex is forged in fantasy. Some have said that a great sex life depends upon a great fantasy life. Justin Lehmiller, author of the book *Tell Me What You Want*, reports that 97 percent of Americans fantasize about sex. How the mental informs the physically sexual and vice versa is complicated. Some people tell themselves they are in love in order to have fulfilling sexual experiences – are they in love? Does it matter what they tell themselves? People may have difficulties having sex when they are angry at each other – why? Are there differences between people who can have sex while angry with their partners and those that cannot? Sex and sexuality raise many difficult but interesting questions.

This complex interaction between the psychological and the physical seems to start when sexual desire begins. At puberty, sex seems often to carry with it the baggage of insecurity. Am I sexually attractive? Are my breasts/penis large enough? Am I more attractive than the other boys or girls? How do I know if I am a good kisser? These mental gymnastics associated with sex begin at puberty and last most of our lives. Even when partnered as adults, people frequently have doubts revolving around sex. Am I still sexy to my significant other? Is my sex life as exciting as that of my friends? Would having a more athletic or thinner body mean better sex? Do I perform as well sexually as my best friends? Do I get as much sex as my best friends, and even the "average" person?

Why does something as rewarding and enjoyable as sex seem to produce such insecurities? Why do people always seem to have so many questions about sex? In part, we struggle with understanding sex due to its very importance for most of us: it is hard to view sex through an objective or impassionate lens. We also have questions about sex because we rarely get any good answers. Although the vast majority of parents would like to have sexual education in schools, only 38 percent of US high schools and 14 percent of middle schools teach all 19 of the sexual health topics considered essential by the Centers for Disease Control (e.g. how to create and sustain healthy and respectful relationships, information on how sexually transmitted infections are spread, and tips about ways partners can communicate to prevent pregnancies or infections). Additionally, in the USA, only 24 states mandate sex education in schools, and of those, only 10 require that it be medically accurate. Despite the all-pervasive nature of sex in modern society, people in school may learn very little about sex and much of it may be inaccurate. That leaves educating to the family, but many families seldom discuss it openly – sex is taboo. Sexual attitudes for many people are therefore mainly sculpted implicitly – rather than through open discussion and objectivity. Research has shown, for example, that age of first sexual experience is heavily influenced by norms and expectations shown by our parents, and next most important is what we "perceive" as being normal in our peer group and culture. Wider cultural norms have been shown to be important across many countries. How well we can control our urges or impulses also plays a role in age at first sexual experience: difficulty regulating behavior, referred to as "impulsivity," is not only associated with earlier sexual activities but also with riskier sexual activities. As we will see throughout this book, apart from some key research groups and research papers, sexual norms and the nature of sexuality have received very little objective research attention.

How much do we know about sex? Most of us had some lectures in high school about sexual health, but it was generally about safe sex, pregnancy, and perhaps sexually transmitted diseases. It almost never addresses questions of sexual desire, and so most people have very little information to use to understand their own behavior or the behaviors of their loved ones. It is also striking that although we may have discussions about sex with friends or partners, those discussions rarely include detailed knowledge about sexual desire. Instead, we rely on others' opinions and what they have heard or read in magazines, either as rumor or as mistruth.

If we know so little about sex, how do we know if and when sexual desire is typical or healthy? Obviously, sexual desire exists along a spectrum. Not everyone has the same level of desire. Part of the problem is that people do not feel comfortable talking about sex, even to intimate partners. In fact, a recent survey found that approximately 30 percent of adults feel uncomfortable talking about sex with their partners, despite having sex frequently. For those who do talk about sex, couples may wait an average of 5 months into the relationship before actively discussing sex and desires. Approximately 20 percent reported that they would never bring up the topic of sex during a relationship.

As practicing psychiatrists who also undertake research, we find that among our patients, individuals can be far more comfortable talking about their sex lives with us, compared with discussing sex with their partner of many years. People who enjoy sex a lot often feel like there is something wrong with them, whereas those who are less interested in sex may feel emasculated or prudish if they admit it. Among our patients, we find that education about sexual desire makes it easier for people to talk openly about their level of desire; talking about desire is the first step in working out what is normal and healthy for the individual, and whether a problem exists for which the person might need support, or even treatment.

Talking about sex is also problematic for many people as they regard the topic as deeply personal. One of us once asked several friends about details of their sex lives. These were close friends with whom he had experienced many emotional situations – loss of parents, serious health concerns such as human immunodeficiency virus (HIV) and cancer, loss of jobs, and divorce. Surprisingly, most of them felt uncomfortable disclosing the sexual details of their lives. Although we know that talking about sex to your friends can potentially be a great way to destigmatize a normal and healthy part of life and shift the conversation about sex from dirty to empowering, only some men and women feel comfortable doing so. The point here is not to be prurient but to shed light on the idea that although sex is hugely important to people, most are unwilling to discuss it, or at least to discuss it in a legitimate or direct fashion. Therefore, we are often left to our own devices, trying to navigate what is or is not healthy or "normal" about our sexual desires. Why, if sex is so important to most of us, and critical for continuation of our species, do many of us have difficulties being open about the topic? We all recognize that we are sexual beings, surrounded by other sexual beings, and yet are often deeply ashamed of being such or of thinking about friends or family in these ways. Why?

One reason for some hesitancy in discussing sex, as well as for the limited available information about sex for most people, is that sex is the one health topic that is deeply entwined with culture and religion/morality/spirituality. Unlike other psychological issues, the way many perceive sex is from the perspective of their cultural or religious upbringing. The problem is that culture and religion may produce messages about sex that differ from those of psychology and science, or messages that can be reconciled but only with much thought. If my sexual desires differ from what my culture teaches me, how do I reconcile that? How do I understand healthy sexual desire given that inconsistency? What does this mean for my sexual relationships with others?

One other cultural value that often gets confused in discussions of sex is that of love. As with all animals, we generally have strong biological drives for sex. Do we have a similar drive for love? Is it the same drive biologically? Some people use sex to get love; others use love to get sex. Couples who have been together for many years may say that they have a strong love keeping them together but that sex has waned. Other couples may fall out of love and still have strong sexual drives for each other. Does that suggest any problems in the relationship?

Independent of culture, religion, or love, some people objectively have atypical levels of sexual desire, either far too low or too high, which feels out of control and leads to unwanted consequences. Either extreme (loss of interest in sex, or excessive preoccupation with sex) may suggest a mental health disorder. Some people have little or no sexual desire, and this may cause problems with relationships and self-esteem. However, it is increasingly recognized that sexual behavior has the potential to become addictive. Just as substances such as alcohol and narcotics are rewarding and habit forming, so too is sex. For these people, a once relatively benign behavior can escalate, leading them to spend inordinate amounts of time preparing for or engaging in sex, meanwhile neglecting other areas of life. People who develop a sexual addiction often experience a great deal of emotional distress, including guilt and shame. What happens to a person that results in them losing their sexual drive? Conversely, how is it possible that sexual behavior can become out of control?

All of these topics of sex may become important for partners, family, and friends. When people learn about others' sexual desires, they may not know how to respond or cope. Partners, parents, and adult children can have a profound sense of helplessness in watching a loved one struggle with issues of sexual desire and may feel implicated in those struggles. For example, if a man finds that his sexual desires are greatly diminished due to health problems, he may feel guilty about being less involved sexually with his wife, and she may interpret his behavior as rejection. Adult children – or a nursing home – may fail to see the importance of sexual companionship for elderly couples. In many situations, loved ones do not know how to help and may even make matters worse.

Sex can be difficult for people to understand. People can easily have sex but have no true understanding of sex. As we will explain later in this book, research has demonstrated the physical basis of sexual desire in the brain. Yet people struggle with the issues of character and morality involved in sexual behavior. As we will explore in more detail, sex is complex. More and more people are discussing their sexual issues with healthcare workers in clinical settings, but they have problems discussing it with others. Unfortunately, many healthcare providers have little background in sexual behavior. Therefore, the Internet is being used to educate people about sex, often with disastrous results. Witness, for example, the recent idea that exposure to large amounts of internet pornography in young people is leading to insecurities about their bodies, unrealistic expectations of sexual experiences, or even impotence as real-life experiences do not live up to the pornography movie they watched.

In our experience of treating patients, we have seen that sexual behavior can be the most important aspect of life and simultaneously the most distressing area of life. We wrote this book with a view to educating people about sex, as well as their partners, relatives, and friends. The book is written to address questions about sex that researchers, clinicians, and members of the public often have but seldom feel comfortable asking anyone about. It considers the latest scientific evidence including from the neurosciences (brain sciences). We hope it will be of interest to members of the public, as well as to a variety of professionals, including those teaching others about these topics (e.g. counselors, social workers, and other educators).

The book begins by outlining what is meant by "desire" and describing how sexual desire is similar and different to other desires. In the next chapters, we consider different topics relevant to sex such as development, healthy sexual behavior in adulthood, and problems with too little or too much sexual desire. There is a chapter on how digital technology has radically changed sex and desire in the last 30 years. There is a chapter examining diverse aspects of sex with a focus on neglected minority groups, as well as cross-cultural perspectives. The book also has a chapter providing practical, step-by-step advice on various problems encountered in relationships due to sexual issues. Lastly, we include a chapter that addresses how times of national crisis have affected sex, including examples of the COVID-19 pandemic and world wars. All these chapters include anonymous, real-life case examples of people with various sexual issues based on our extensive clinical practice (details about these people have been modified, left out, or distorted to maintain strict confidentiality). At the end of the book, you will find a list of resources around the world for people with these behaviors who are seeking more information or treatment. We also list some further reading on each topic, as we are aware that no single book can address all of the issues of a very complex topic.

Above all, we wrote this book because, although much is known about sex, little information is available for those who want a detailed discussion of a variety of topics associated with sexual desire. We hope this text will help to inform others about sex based on the latest scientific evidence, get people thinking about the complexity of this common behavior, and encourage new research to address the important knowledge gaps that exist in this area.

2   Sex and Desire

Susan is a 42-year-old single woman who enjoys sex and dates fairly frequently. She has found that over the years, she has become less interested in marriage and more interested in having a fulfilling sexual life. She feels comfortable with her body, has confidence in her career and her identity, and wants to be able to have fun with men. For her, sex is a large part of that fun. Susan also feels that she now channels some of her work desires into her personal life. Successful in business, she now spends time in the evening dating and going out, and less time thinking of ways of making larger profits for her business. She exercises a few hours each day and has watched her diet. She feels these go together somehow – exercise, sex, dieting, and her work ethic; as one rises as a priority, another may fall a bit. Friends have commented that this new insistence on sex and dating is unlike her former self, but Susan feels that she is the same person, simply shifting priorities.

Patrick is a 28-year-old male who enjoys dating and sex but sees sex as a means of forming a relationship with a woman. In fact, he feels his strongest desire is for love and that sex is important but secondary to love. He does admit that he often fools himself into believing he is in love because he wants sex and feels guilty having sex without loving the person. Patrick has issues with his body and feels he is not particularly good at sex. Also, the women he enjoys in pornography are not the types of women he would want to date, but he wishes the women he dates could be more sexual like those in pornography. Patrick reports having dated some women who wanted sex much more frequently than he did and he felt inadequate as he could not get as interested in sex as they were. He also feels that the sexual imbalance may have ultimately ruined the relationships.

Sexual desire is hugely important to most people, but it can also be time consuming, and frustrating. Religion, politics, philosophy, psychology, and neuroscience have all attempted to understand, explain, and even control sexual desire. This chapter explores the complex topic of sexual desire and its relationship to other desires of appetite. Understanding what is arguably meant by healthy desire may allow us to explain and possibly address instances where our desires become less healthy or more problematic.

Desire

The concept of desire is multiplex. On a simple level, the term desire refers to wanting something. But even wanting something is not simple, and there may be varying degrees of wanting. There are also multiple domains of desire, and in fact philosophy has written about desire for centuries (e.g. longing for purpose, desire for resources). In this chapter, we are interested in desire for all kinds of pleasure, including closeness, intimacy, beauty, family, and friendship, as well as sex. Why do we desire something or someone? Do we or can we really know why? Our development, our current state of life, our peer group, and our future dreams, both real and imaginary, all seem to factor into what we desire and how intensely we desire it.

The Purpose of Sexual Desire

Sexual desire serves many purposes. First, there is a simple evolutionary reason for desire and that is procreation. Of course, reproduction does not require sex, and in fact sex may have drawbacks (e.g. only half of an individual's genes are passed on to each offspring, and courtship and mating are risky). Sexual reproduction, however, may purge genetic mutations and so sexual reproduction tends to be more universal than asexual reproduction. We desire to have our genes spread to future generations and so we have sex.

This seems simple, but why then would gay people have sexual desire? The same reason, probably. The object of desire differs, but the goal may have started the same. But homosexuality doesn't spread genes, and so is there something incompatible between homosexuality and evolution? Some theories posit that being gay is an internal check on population control for all animals. If we have desire, there must be some constraints, otherwise all species might over-breed. Being gay, or the animal version of gay, keeps desire in check and – some argue – directs it for the good of the species. Others suggest a sociosexual hypothesis that human sexuality evolved as humans became more sociable. Thus, the evolution of sex is not only about reproduction but also about social functioning. Same-sex attraction may have evolved because individuals with some degree of same-sex

SEX AND DESIRE

attraction benefited from greater social mobility, integra-
tion, and stronger same-sex social bonds.

Spreading genes does not explain everything about
sexual desire. Related to spreading genes is the need for
survival. Desire can help us survive by keeping us safe and
healthy. We try things in nature to eat, drink, or have sex
with, and the things we enjoy, we do again, whereas we learn
to avoid unpleasant or dangerous things. Rewarding behaviors are reinforced. Of course, these can get out of control if
the reward we feel is particularly intense (see Chapter 6), or
if the reward is associated with one of the dangerous things
of the world – we might strive to do it again and again even
though we know it is damaging for us or for those around us.

Desire itself is a drive state. Intrinsically, it is neither
good nor bad. The objects of desire, however, can be
unhealthy, healthy, or anywhere in between. As our brains
develop during our lives, part of our rational thought process is to understand what a healthy object of desire is, and
how to control ourselves from acting on unhealthy choices.
Full development of these cognitive processes of self-control
(regulation of our urges) often takes until our mid-20s.
Unfortunately, not everyone develops in the same fashion
or at the same pace, or even reaches the same conclusions.
Many life events can alter the development of our desires
and the ability to control them – health issues, early-life
traumatic experiences, drugs and alcohol, and mental illness
can all affect this balance. It also raises the topic of those
people who understand their desires and the healthy choices
and yet choose deliberately not to follow their better judgment. This may have less to do directly with issues in brain

development and more to do with other life issues such as poverty, early-life trauma, and relationship problems.

Imaginative Desires

We all have sexual fantasies. In fact, it is normal, and even healthy, to have sexual fantasies. Imagination plays a vital role in sexual desire and in desire in general. We are able to imagine events in the future, and imagination may enable us to cope with, or escape from, reality. In the realm of the nonsexual, young people spend hours – even years – of hard work desiring certain future imagined paths and yet they do not know what those careers are really like. Those career paths have not yet generated rewards, and so is the imagined outcome what motivates a person in their career goals? This type of desire sounds quite similar to sexual desire for many people.

Imagined desire is quite complicated. The relationship between fantasies (sexual or nonsexual) and reality is complex. Fantasies should be perceived as potentially real so that a person can experience them as credible. The ability to fulfill one's fantasies, however, requires separating oneself from the present reality so as to immerse a person into the excitement of the imagined. Part of the excitement may be a desire to achieve or obtain something that seems valuable to other people, or difficult to get. Desire for many things may also be characterized by the fact that others want it, and therefore I must want it too. The desire is for exclusivity or specialness and perhaps not necessarily the details of the object I am striving for. From this viewpoint, sexual desire may often not be about a pretty face or someone's body but rather a desire to obtain what others desire. In such instances, desire seems to be a desire to win a perceived competition. Therefore, Bill wants to have sex with Sarah, and Michael wants to have sex with Sarah. Bill's desire is really about beating Michael. Interestingly, the focus of Bill's desire is essentially Michael. This highlights the complexity and the focus of desire for any individual, as it is difficult to know when a person has achieved their desire, given that it is not always clear what the true focus of desire is, or its true motivations.

Society's Role in Sexual Desire

In addition to the factors mentioned above, social values and triggers can play a role in the development of our desires. In attempting to explain why we have sexual desire, many people over the years have argued that sexual desire is somehow socially constructed. According to this argument, many aspects of human behavior, including sexual desire, are constructed by the culture in which they exist. People did not smell until someone invented deodorant. That means that until someone created a feeling of "lack", we smelled the same but we did not think we needed anything such as deodorant – we probably did not give Bob's pungent body odor a second thought. Once we lack something, we desire to end that lack or fill that perceived lack. A large part of desire is about perceived needs and what others have. Even some of our "real" needs for sex or food are just perceived desires. For example, we do not need as much food as we often desire. Similarly, we often desire sex when we feel bad about ourselves, but we do not actually need sex. In that case, sometimes our need for sex may perhaps more appropriately be conceived as a desire to be wanted or comforted.

Sexual desire, in particular, seems heavily influenced by social pressures, although this may not mean it is simply a social construct. Sexual desire appears to be deeply biological, and yet social factors elicit desires to varying degrees. One means of doing this is via a focus on body image. Body image is a multidimensional construct, and culturally people from different groups have different body ideals. Regardless of the specific body ideal, however, sexual desire and body image appear to be linked to varying degrees. In the case of blind individuals, aspects of body image such as the texture of skin and hair, smell, and the sound of a voice factor into sexual desire. We sell everything by showing sexy bodies alongside the object we are ostensibly selling, such as a car. We know that desire for the woman's body becomes linked to desire for the car. This also taps into the idea of "lack" that we just discussed. You lack the car and you lack the pretty woman – buy one and get the other as well. Fulfill that lack. Sexual desire is strong and thoughts about sex occupy much of our time, but sexual behavior occupies a small amount of time. A person masturbates or has sex, has an orgasm, and then sex is not much in the thought process for a while. The act of sex is generally a small fraction of our lives in comparison to how much time we work or sleep. By creating social links between sexual desire and the rest of our lives, we become more desirous people. That helps anyone trying to sell us things, because when we desire something strongly, we think less about the consequences or the costs.

Is Sexual Desire the Same as Other Desires?

Throughout this chapter, we have alluded to the idea that there are multiple types of desires, but there may be similarities between the various desires. Humans can obviously become excited and thus desire many rewarding things or behaviors. Sex, eating, drugs, and extreme sports may all tap into the same basic neurobiology of the brain and thereby produce excitement, euphoria, and a need to repeat the behavior. What we have learned from research regarding the treatment of Parkinson's disease is that when the chemical dopamine is revved up in the brain (i.e. through the use of medications that are approved to treat Parkinson's disease), some people can become more desirous of sex, as well as increasing their eating, and even have stronger desires for other rewards such as shopping, gambling, alcohol, and drug use. This suggests that underlying all of these desires, biologically, may be a somewhat similar, or at least overlapping, process or mechanism.

In Chapter 3, we discuss the biological details of sexual desire. So, although desire may have similarities across many rewarding behaviors, it does not stand to reason that sexual desire is simply an identical version of these other appetites of humans.

Sexual desire, like eating or other desires, is also about learned behavior. When we are young, we get cues about what we should desire sexually, both explicitly from family and friends ("She's pretty – you should ask her to dance") but also implicitly from social values and the things we see (e.g. certain body types in advertisements that are attractive, or social constructs of desire such as television shows of houses with white picket fences where pretty people are happy and in love). Research suggests that those with stronger sexual desire have greater incentive motivational processes related to the cues of sex and that certain areas of the brain (anterior cingulate, ventral striatum, and amygdala – areas related to emotional learning, and assigning emotional importance to internal and external stimuli such as images) are overactivated in people with greater sexual desire. Additionally, studies show that we gradually become habituated to sexual cues and so, over time, what we tell ourselves about what excites us will probably chronically excite us due to habit. However, we may also seek out novelty to obtain a higher reward.

When you think about these aspects of sexual desire, doesn't it sound quite like many other desires? For example, there is a lot of learning that informs the development of our food appetites and desires, such as parents telling us what to eat ("That's delicious–try it"), and what we learn about desirable tastes from media and peers ("I would never eat that. It's disgusting and will make you fat"). Habit also plays a role in why we continue to eat and desire certain foods. A good example is beer, often referred to as an acquired taste. We find very few people who have ever liked the taste of beer initially (in fact, the bitterness is often initially off-putting for people). Drinking beer with friends in a bar and having fun, however, creates a context wherein the desire is for the fun and beer comes along eventually for the ride. Over time, people feel the desire for the beer. To some extent, this is mirrored in sexual desire as studies show that many (even most) people really do not enjoy their first sexual experience and yet over time, often due to the context of dating, grow to desire sex.

The Shape of Desire

The above examples highlight two other important aspects of desire. First, although we desire things biologically, we can learn to mold that desire and direct it in many ways, such as learning to desire beer – or avoid it. Can we learn to desire sex in different ways? Yes. Research shows that education is correlated with the extent to which one experiments sexually. In short, those who have more formal education are typically more diversified or more varied in their sex lives. For example, those who go to college are more likely to desire oral sex as part of their sexual repertoire. Is this because education provides greater awareness of the fun or joy of multiple sex acts, or is it a larger issue that education is associated with greater curiosity of the world and that also underlies sex? It could be both. Also, we can change the focus of our desire or expand upon it, but this does not necessarily mean that desire is increased. A person can sexually desire a thing to a great extent and another person may sexually desire a few things to far lesser degrees. This again sounds terribly like food, doesn't it? We expand our appetites via education and exposure to new things (e.g. I never ate Japanese food until college and thought it was amazing). We do not necessarily increase the intensity of our overall food desire though.

The second point from the link between sex and food suggests that the context in which we experience a reward may be as much a part of the desire as the actual object itself. Romantic restaurants for a first date, a Hawaiian vacation setting where we meet someone – these become part of the sexual desire that we feel for that person. This is a consequence of associative learning: the brain learns to link particular settings and contexts with reward. Context can also be about risk and excitement, such as sex in a public place with a stranger. The context may increase the reward value and that will in turn create desire for the reward again. Similarly, in a food-related example, we might desire a buckwheat scone but only when we imagine getting it from a specific coffee shop, at a particular time of day. We might never make or eat the scone at home, even though it would be fairly easy to do so. We desire certain foods but only at certain restaurants. We simply do not have the same desire for them outside a particular context. In these cases, does the person desire the object or the "package" of the object in a certain context? Could it be both?

Families Matter in Our Desires

In both of the above situations, you can also see that developmental issues such as how we are raised can shape our initial desires, whether good or bad. We can obviously be educated about desire and have desires expand, but we often hold very strong beliefs about desire – how strong it should be and where it should be directed – based on our upbringing. Several systematic reviews have demonstrated that parents play a key role in shaping their children's views about sexual behavior and ultimately their decision making throughout the adolescent years. The evidence also demonstrates that many parents underestimate their role in teaching their children about sex. As a result, many adolescents report little or no communication about sex with their parents. Given that few young people are fully educated at home about sexual desire, this may explain the benefits of sexual education in schools. Evidence-based sexual health education can actually improve academic success, prevent dating violence and bullying, help youth develop healthier relationships, reduce unplanned pregnancies and sexually transmitted diseases, and reduce sexual health disparities among LGBTQ (lesbian, gay, bisexual, transgender, queer) youth.

Should Desire Be Acted Upon or Suppressed?

People grapple with their desires, often due to conflicts or mismatches between what they desire and their family values or their own values. For example, research from the US Centers for Disease Control and Prevention (CDC) suggests that when adolescents speak to their parents about sex, the topic is usually either how to say "no" to sex or about sexually transmitted diseases, both of which may in turn be more about suppressing sexual desire. Oscar Wilde wrote that the only way to resist temptation was to yield to it. This is obviously witty but not useful advice in all situations. Desires that are socially prohibited or problematic for someone else should probably not be acted upon. In other situations, we may act on a desire when we balance the strength of the desire against the possible dangers of the desire. If our internal calculations are in favor of the desire, we act on it. In fact, that sort of decision-making process underlies almost every choice we make, even if we are not always aware of doing the calculations. In the case of adolescent sexual desire, however, parents and educators become vital players in balancing the dangers of desire with the urges (adolescents may simply be unable to fully understand the medium- to longer-term effects of their decisions).

It is possible that acting on a desire may make the behavior more intensely desired the next time. Sex and food are again good examples as they share these qualities. If a person has great sex with someone they know is not a healthy partner psychologically, the desire to have further great sex may override reservations concerning the person's character. This is opposed to simply resisting the desire and letting it naturally burn out. Similarly, eating something high in fat that tastes good may make a person crave it again, whereas if resisted, they may forget about it and never want it again.

People differ quite a bit in these respects and so there is no rule of thumb. Some people report that if they get a taste of their desired object, they can stop the behavior. They seem to have great inner strength and control. Other people report that any taste of something makes them want lots more of whatever it is – that they have an "addictive personality." In the case of desire for drugs and alcohol, this may be why some people can drink or use drugs responsibly while others drink to intoxication every time they touch liquor.

Complicating this picture have been recent advances in neurosciences that show that if a person thinks about doing something quite seriously and in detail, the brain registers it as if the person actually did it (at least to a major extent). Indeed, this has led to new neuroimaging tests that can detect consciousness in people who were thought to be in a vegetative state. This knowledge has also been used to good effect in competitive sports with the notion that performance can be improved over time by visualizing one's self doing the sport. This is interesting and mirrors old teachings in some religions that thinking is the same as doing. Nuns might tell us as a child that if we had a bad thought it was the same as doing the wicked deed. This idea also differs from the legal world (thank goodness) wherein we can think about all sorts of terrible things and not get into legal trouble, but if we did the same things, we would have major problems. But assuming for some people, who consider things in exquisite detail, that thinking is registered in the brain the same as doing, should they avoid even thinking about the desire or suppress the thoughts? Not all thoughts lead to actions, and so it probably differs from person to person. This ability for thoughts not to translate into acts may have a substantial amount to do with other variables in the brain, such as the circuits involved in controlling or inhibiting behavior. If those cir-cuits are strong, then thoughts are just thoughts and most likely will not lead to actions. Also, it is quite common to experience thoughts that psychiatrists call "egodystonic" – this means that the thoughts are not consistent with who we are or what we want to do.

Directing or Restraining Desire

Context can make a desire acceptable or unacceptable. On a Friday evening at a bar or club, we can allow desire to flourish. On a Monday morning at the office, desire is less acceptable. We may have intimate relationships with our partner 3 days a week, often on the same days or times of day. Many of us relegate desire to certain times and contexts. In fact, surveys of married couples have found that a majority of people schedule their sexual activities.

Context may also help to limit or restrain desire. Relegating desire to certain days and times may work to put restraints on desire and make us more productive at other times. It is a bit like the theory that weekends allow larger social desires to play out so that we are all more productive for the rest of the week. If we desire something or someone all the time, then we might never be productive, and hedonism would reign. That might be fun, but we would never get the laundry done. Some people believe that they should not act on sexual desire if they want to be successful in their careers. There is no evidence that desire is a limited or finite quantity in any one person. It makes sense that a person can have sexual desire and desire for a career as well. Time might be the rate-limiting step in trying to do everything but not desire.

In these cases, where the context drives some of the desire, does it do a disservice to the person who may be the object of desire? If the neighborhood bar on Friday evening has made me randy, is it less flattering to the object of my desire when we are intimate on a Friday after meeting at the bar? Was it the bar or the person who triggered my desire? Obviously, there is no easy answer to this as it may change based on the person and even within the same person given different evenings. What it does suggest is that desire comes from many areas, and we may not be consciously aware of how much triggers our desires when we ask someone home on a Friday evening at a bar.

If Desire Becomes "Habit," Can We Lose Desire?

Some of the previous discussion has suggested that context as a trigger for desire may, over time, reduce the intensity of desire as it becomes habitual. This most likely depends upon the person. For those who enjoy novelty, the idea of habit may quickly reduce the intensity of desire. For those who crave predictability and comfort, desire may be further intensified by having the habit of context drive our desires. Knowing these aspects of ourselves might be important before acting on desire. The person who likes novelty may need a very different sexual arrangement in life than the person who craves predictability. This could be differences in the variety of sexual activities or in the exclusivity of their partners or marriage, for example. Knowing who we are versus who we wish we were could be handy before launching into relationships that do not fit well with our underlying personality type. For example, for a young man who loves excitement and novelty, it may be uncomfortable getting married young and living in the suburbs with the white picket fence, even if he wishes he were the type of man who could do that.

Desire and Deceit

We have noticed in our clinical practices that people lie, and one area that people lie the most about is desire. This can be lying about how much they eat or how frequently they get intoxicated, as well as what they desire sexually. It is partly due to embarrassment that people lie (they do not want to admit what they have desired or if they have acted on desire to an unhealthy extent) and possibly due to control (a fundamental human belief is that we are in control of our behavior). People lie to their intimate partners as well as lying to themselves. We find that most people probably have little idea about the sexual desires of the person they are partnered with. This has been a troubling revelation for us over the years as we see so many people who live two lives – the one for their partners and another one that is secretive. This happens in people of all classes, education levels, races/ethnicities, and professions. These people often have wonderful lives, at least on the surface. From our perspective, getting to know people initially produced some cynicism about love and desire and the idea that they were so divorced from complete honesty and veracity. Over time, however, we have grown to accept the idea that desire leads to dishonesty and incompleteness (i.e. not telling or exposing the entire person) not because people are bad or deceptive but because desire is so powerful and at times all-consuming that people feel out of control about it. This lack of control, both consciously and unconsciously, leads to attempts to take control of one's primal self and one's life by lying.

Mystery is alluring. Therefore, the irony is that lying may even lead to increased sexual desire. Lying to a partner now casts a behavior as naughty or secretive. This may in turn make the behavior more rewarding and thereby desirable. So, desire often leads to lying, which leads to more desire. The problem is that this may be fine if a person exists in a vacuum, but when someone else is involved in the relationship, the lying can ultimately be destructive.

Summary

This chapter has described the complex concept of desire, what generates drive and why, and how the idea of desire might apply to drives other than sex. The case of Susan highlights the idea that desire may be a universal drive with different foci but a common drive informed by learned behavior, biological necessities, and social pressures. Patrick's story adds an additional layer of complexity to the story of desire, as love may be an additional variable or at least a variable that a person overlays on desire to explain a drive that is often out of one's control to understand. These areas will be explored further in the following chapters.

3   Development Issues around Sex

Joanne is a 13-year-old school student. Mr. Jones, a newly qualified history teacher, has recently started working at the school. Joanne's female friends point out that they find Mr. Jones attractive, and they engage in sex talk about him, fantasizing about situations and wondering whether he is married. He is debonair and physically attractive. Joanne gets red-faced and embarrassed in front of her friends when they talk about this. She has developed a crush on Mr. Jones and has recently started masturbating about him. She wonders if the crush is normal, as it hasn't happened before. Joanne feels incredibly guilty about masturbating and feels she is doing something wrong or unnatural; there is no way she would be able to speak to anyone about this.

As explored in the Chapter 2, desire refers to our wants and cravings throughout life. Far from being consistent in nature and intensity, our desires change over the course of our lifespan – and can even, sometimes, switch on or off overnight. Our conscious mind or "ego" cannot always control our desires; in contrast, we are very good at using our intellect to feed or achieve our desires, whether for good or ill. The above case vignette leads us to think about how desire for sex develops over the lifespan, and what is "normal."

Animal Drive

Desire is a powerful way of motivating behavior. The simplest type of animal on Earth – an amoeba – is made up of just one self-contained cell. It is amazing to think that amoebae, despite their simplicity, are able to move around and eat, by moving finger-like projections. We are not suggesting that amoeba experience the richness of experiences and flexible behavior that more complicated animal species can – they do not even have a "brain." But what this demonstrates is that even ancient animal life, from the perspective of evolution, developed mechanisms to navigate the environment and obtain what they need – and, ultimately, what they want (which often is not the same thing). If a simple animal species was suddenly dropped onto an empty planet through a mysterious force, members of that species who had some desire versus no desire would quickly take over. But there can be costs to being built with a predisposition for desire, as this book will explore in some detail.

Desire is fundamental to human existence – without any desire, we would not eat, drink, move, or procreate. Say goodbye to us and our potential offspring! But it is not enough just to have desire. To be efficient, we need some common mechanism or brain "circuitry" for experiencing desire and then implementing actions from it. Nature likes efficiency – using the smallest possible amount of resources (energy) to achieve the most beneficial outcome. It would not make evolutionary sense for us to develop separate brain circuits to fuel our desire for fat, sugar, chocolate, sex, love, procreation, holidays, and a host of other desires that can help us survive and perhaps live a fulfilling existence. William of Ockham was an English friar who is attributed with the principle of "Occam's razer." This principle says that if there are many different scientific hypotheses, the one with fewest assumptions should usually be chosen, because there are thousands – potentially infinitely – more complicated models that could be developed to explain a concept. It is more efficient to choose the simpler model. Nature tends to follow this principle: simplicity and common biological mechanisms to achieve a goal are best, because they are more resource efficient. It makes sense that our brains would have common pathways through which we experience markedly different types of desire and translate those desires into actions.

Desire and the Brain

Desire rests in our brains. The brain is an incredibly complex organism – the average adult brain has 86 billion neurons or cells, and 1000 trillion synaptic connections (connections between neurons). Cells communicate with each other through chemical messengers called neurotransmitters, which include dopamine, norepinephrine, serotonin, and a host of others. Over time, our brains change and remodel extensively – from birth through childhood, puberty, and adulthood, through to middle age and older age. There are structural changes to the tissue: some neurons die in a planned way, some form more connections, and others shed their connections with other neurons. This is called structural plasticity or remodeling. Brains also show functional plasticity – the strength of different connections changes, along with the levels of neurotransmitters – rather akin to a computer that can change not only its own hardware but also its software. These structural and functional changes in the brain help us to adapt flexibly to different environments and different roles in society, and also to changes in our body such as those during puberty. As we will see later, profound changes in *what* we desire, and *how* we desire, come about because of this plasticity.

The brain has a common pathway for desire. Evolutionarily, the ancient parts of the brain that play a key role in desire are the ventral tegmentum and nucleus accumbens, which are important clusters of nerve cells. When the ventral tegmentum and nucleus accumbens are stimulated by titillating information from our sensory organs (e.g. seeing someone we fancy, smelling a voluptuous meal, or being stroked), we experience pleasure. Activation of the ventral tegmentum causes dopamine to be released in the nucleus accumbens and frontal cortex. In parallel, another "reward" neurotransmitter – glutamate – is released in the nucleus accumbens. Consuming drugs with addictive potential, such as alcohol or nicotine, leads to pleasurable experiences because these drugs (or chemical by-products of these drugs) cross into the central nervous system and hijack this desire circuitry temporarily. Over time, if we keep using addictive drugs, the versatile brain learns to activate the desire pathway not only through direct effects of the drug but also by environmental cues (e.g. smelling something we associate with the drug, such as the odor of tobacco). Hence, perceiving these cues tells the desire pathway, "Hey, this is something worth looking into! Why not find someone with a spare cigarette and smoke?" Similarly, as we will see in Chapter 6, repeated sexual activity for some individuals can become addictive: "Hey! I get a massive reward from hooking up in this club – I'll go there again."

Control over Desire

If we desire to eat chocolate, and we eat the chocolate, we experience a reward. What stops us (or at least, most of us – except chocoholics) from then immediately eating chocolate again, getting more reward, and repeating the process over and over – a loop of infinite chocoholism? This could also happen for sex – we indulge in a sexual activity and it is rewarding, so why don't most of us repeat it over and over forever, ignoring other aspects of our life, especially when sex can be so intrinsically and acutely rewarding? This loss of control does happen for some people, leading to what might be referred to as a pathological habit or behavioral addiction. We will discuss more about when desire gets out of control in Chapter 6. The answer to this conundrum is that the brain has a specific mechanism – a "brake" – that has developed to prevent such a thing happening to us, to prevent one rewarding habit taking control over our lives.

It is the more recently evolved parts of the brain that are important in our brain's brake system. In the frontal lobes sit the inferior frontal gyrus and orbitofrontal gyrus, containing neurons responsible for regulating our behavioral responses to desire. When these regions are damaged, such as from trauma or tumors, people who were previously reserved and not very preoccupied with their desires may run amok with desire, becoming sexually disinhibited, spending money recklessly, saying hurtful things to people they care about, or even being violent to those they love. Their personality can radically change overnight. This happens because the regions responsible for stopping our urges and impulses have stopped working. If other regions of the cortex are damaged to a similar extent, the ability to control responses to desire is barely affected, but of course there could be other problems depending on the role of the affected region – such as in memory, attention, our ability to plan things ahead of time, or in being able to speak or interpret words we hear.

The inferior frontal and orbitofrontal cortex brake regions can also be knocked out of action temporarily rather than permanently, through consuming drugs such as alcohol. When we get intoxicated or "high," chemical signaling in these brake regions can be disrupted by the substances we have taken, leading to desires that would normally be suppressed or stilted coming out. Visit the emergency room of any hospital on a Friday night and you will see carnage resulting from the negative effects of drugs on our brain's natural brake system. Alcohol contributes to fights, road traffic accidents, impulsive sex, and other ills. Many of us have done things we later regretted while under the influence of alcohol – not necessarily to the above degree – but typically more during our youth than in our later adulthood. Chronic alcohol use, or use of other drugs, can even affect the structure and function of these brain pathways in a more persisting way that is harder to reverse.

Why are young people more prone to giving in to their desires, when confronted with them? Why is there such a term as "youthful indiscretion"? The reason is that the brain's brake systems, just like the brain's desire system, is not cast in stone before birth but undergoes changes through development. Brain imaging studies have found that the brain's brake system develops during adolescence but does not fully mature until our late 20s, or even later than that, into our 30s. In contrast, our desire system seems to show the main plastic changes during adolescence and settles down around then. The net effect is that adolescence is a time when we are seething with desire but have yet to develop the biological mechanisms to dampen them down as an older adult would. It follows that young people are quite vulnerable to peer pressure and hedonistic traps of taking cocktails of drugs or spending recklessly. While such behaviors can develop at any age, adolescence is often the first time we are primed for certain desires (those that are sexual) or exposed to them more fully (availability of alcohol and drugs). We start to mix socially outside our family circle, to gain more independence, and we are more exposed to people and situations that can involve sexual activity.

The Complicated Brake System of the Brain

The decision to act on a particular craving or desire can be entirely positive in the moment, but the consequences could be negative. The chain of positives and negatives can be very complicated. Humans are uniquely situated in the animal kingdom in terms of being able to think ahead of time about the future consequence of our short-term more immediate actions. An individual looking at a tempting piece of chocolate might think, "It costs me no effort to eat the chocolate – and it's just one chocolate, so it won't affect my weight." True, but what if the individual had worked hard to lose weight previously? They might have learned that keeping chocolate at home was a bad idea in the first place; and they might – in the moment of seeing the chocolate – recollect the previous effort it took to lose weight and how unhappy they felt when they were larger. Our ability to resist urges is colored by our previous experiences and by our conscious mind, which can reason through sequences of possibilities and emotional memory. An ex-smoker might learn to avoid work meals out at the bar, because – based on past experience – she knows that these events would involve exposure to the smell of cigarette smoke, and then that she would almost certainly be unable to resist smoking. A businessman offered the prospect of anonymous sex at an international conference, with a wife at home, might turn it down despite extremely strong desire – even if the chance of his partner finding out was essentially zero – out of love or a sense of morality. Our efforts to resist desire stem from a host of complex other emotions and past learning experiences, so while the origin of desire and the ability to suppress responses lie within the brain, it does not follow that they are simple to understand or straightforward.

Sexual Awakening: Early Sexual Desire

In the case example of Joanne, the 13-year-old girl who developed a crush on her new history teacher, she is experiencing a sexual awakening. This means a growing awareness of one's own body functions related to sex and also finding others, or even objects or situations, sexually appealing. Sexual awakening is almost universally a difficult and awkward period of development. Despite the all-pervasive nature of sex on our television screens, in our newspapers, and on the Internet, society is surprisingly coy at discussing sexual desire. There are hundreds of terms for masturbation in men such as "spanking the monkey" or "charming the snake," which serve to humorize but also to avoid directly discussing the topic. It is perhaps informative about society that such common terms do not exist for masturbation in women, despite a considerable proportion of women engaging in masturbation, albeit not as commonly as men. Other aspects related to sex are alluded to in conversations rather than spoken about directly; examples include stories about the "birds and the bees," or babies being made in a "cabbage patch" or dropped off by a stork. Yes, these are stories told to children, but they are also used in adulthood again to humorize but also reflecting embarrassment. We are sure you can think of other examples.

As young people enter puberty, signaling the beginning of adolescence, a host of changes occur in the body. By sexual awakening, we refer to puberty and changes that happen in the body and brain during this time, not necessarily sexual intercourse itself. The different hormone systems kick into action, triggering chemical cascades, the end products of which include increased levels of testosterone and estrogen. In turn, these chemical cascades cause rapid changes in physical appearance – we grow taller, our facial shape changes, and we develop sexual characteristics (e.g. hair growth, development of breast tissue in women, and enlargement of the voice box in men). Importantly, there are large changes not only to the body in adolescence but also to the brain. The brain feeds back via signaling pathways to the body, and the body feeds back via signaling pathways to the brain, to prepare us for becoming sexual beings. The changes in testosterone and estrogen levels have a direct effect on the desire circuits of the brain, sensitizing the nucleus accumbens and parts of the cortex (including the frontal lobe and visual cortex) to respond to sex-relevant information from the external world, such as seeing breasts or muscular bodies. There are additional changes in other brain regions, including the hypothalamus, which makes us more primed – more likely – to engage in sex-relevant activities.

Faced with this gradual and complicated switch from nonsexual beings to sexually interested beings, adolescents face a steep learning curve, and the brain continues to be plastic and to adapt. It is early during this adolescent period that many adolescents experience one or more "crushes" like Joanne – sexual desire or obsessiveness toward an individual that is typically one-sided, unrealistic, temporary, and not reciprocated. Early in puberty, a given individual would be fertile – capable of fathering or giving birth to offspring. Just because someone is capable of having children, does not mean that they attempt to do so. Sexual awakening is not just about sex. Humans have a complex repertoire of sex-relevant behaviors and we also develop rich fantasy lives about sex, which can be entirely disconnected from reality. Teenagers engage in a variety of behaviors that are sex-relevant. This includes simply learning to communicate with people we are interested in, in terms of both verbal language and also body language. In nearly all societies, adolescents are theoretically capable of sex and procreation – on average – several years before society would regard sexual activity as acceptable for that age. Just because an adolescent is theoretically capable of sex and procreation does not mean they will necessarily engage in sexual intercourse around that time, because there are important factors molding behavior beyond simple biology, such as the societal and parental norms discussed in Chapter 2.

Sexual Awakening in Boys and Girls

The average onset of puberty, defined in terms of development of sexual characteristics and activation of the hormone systems described above, is different between the sexes. Boys tend to enter puberty between 11 and 12 years of age, whereas girls start at 10–11 years old (although there are many exceptions to these general averages). There is also growing evidence that in Western cultures the age of starting puberty has been getting younger over the years. There is also some evidence in the USA that the age of puberty onset differs based on race; for example, Black men start puberty a year younger than White men. The reasons for this earlier age of puberty or the influence of race are still unknown. People have suggested multiple theories such as increased body mass index in children, and nutritional factors or hormonal influences in dietary intake, but there has been no clear cause.

There are other sex differences regarding starting puberty and becoming sexual beings. If a girl gets pregnant, she and her family are left handling the dramatic life-changing consequences. If a boy gets a girl pregnant, there are consequences but certainly not of the life-changing degree that the girl would have to contend with. Society's attitude toward sex is different between the sexes and this has been discussed for decades. Females are brought up to value their modesty – to put it directly, limiting sexual activity to few or no partners, unless in the context of a longer-term partnership. In addition, young women are often taught to attend to others' needs, avoid conflict, and be hyperattentive to their physical appearance. Society, in contrast, often encourages males to be sexual – a man or teenaged boy who engages in a sexual experience is commonly socially elevated among his male peers, whereas a women or teenaged girl who does so is more commonly admonished in her peer group and spoken about in pejorative terms, or even cast out of her peer group completely. In some cultural settings in certain countries, women have even been imprisoned or killed due to perceived unsanctioned sexual activity, even by members of their own family, whereas this would seldom happen to boys.

In adolescence, most males have their first experience of sexual pleasure through masturbation (because this is more common in men; across all age groups, approximately 70 percent of men compared to 50 percent of women masturbate), whereas for many women, the first sexual experience is in the context of activities with another person. Why is there a difference in rates of masturbation between the sexes? There may be multiple influences on why boys masturbate more than girls. Studies in primates suggest that regular masturbation may maintain semen and sperm quality. Access to information about masturbation, hormonal differences, and the respective anatomical differences between males and females may all play a role. Importantly, there are often cultural and social influences that condone male sexual expressions and suppress female sexuality. Interestingly, research shows that healthcare providers usually omit any discussion of masturbation; in a study where 64 percent of parents with children aged 12 years or older recalled discussions with their healthcare provider on sexuality, only 6 percent of discussions addressed masturbation.

Partly because of this difference in rates of masturbation, but also because of other reasons including the different social attitudes toward the genders, young men tend to think about relationships in terms of sex, while women tend to think more in terms of mutual activities, bonding, and conversation. As we get older, these discrepancies become blurred so that men and women are more similar in attitudes. This partly reflects differences in the onset and speed of development between men and women.

First Sexual Intercourse and Its Public Health Importance

Why are public health professionals so preoccupied with teenage sexual intercourse? The reason is that an earlier age of first sexual experience correlates strongly with risks of unplanned pregnancy and spreading of sexually transmitted disease. Younger people are less likely to use condoms and other forms of contraception consistently. Younger people may also lack experience of how to use contraceptive methods effectively. There is also a higher risk of exploitation through violent or unbalanced relationships in people who have earlier first sexual experiences. Earlier sexual experience has been linked with doing less well in education and in terms of employment, in the longer term. Adolescents are especially vulnerable to impulsive sexual acts because the brain's brake system is less well developed than that of older people, they have less experience with which to judge decisions and others' intentions, and, at this sensitive time, peer pressure can be especially overwhelming.

The age when people first have different types of first sexual experiences, including sexual intercourse, varies considerably between individuals, generations, and cultural settings. In the USA, the majority of individuals report their first sexual intercourse before the age of 20 years. If one considers previous generations, the age of initial sexual activity tended to be older due to different attitudes and norms; over time, the trend has been toward a younger age at first sexual experience, a fact that is concerning because the brake system – as we noted – of younger people's brains is less developed. This makes risky sexual activities, on average, more likely (e.g. not using a condom, leading to early pregnancies and spread of sexually transmitted infections). In cultures where sex before marriage – or outside of marriage – is regarded as unacceptable, the average age of the first sexual experience has shown the opposite trend, increasing over time, because people are getting married at older ages than was historically the case, and marriage is the primary setting for sex.

What specific factors in the environment might be responsible for affecting whether someone has sexual activity at a younger age than they would do otherwise? An earlier age of first sexual experience is associated with less parental supervision, less chance of parents teaching their children about sex within a moral and/or religious framework, and more peer pressure. Schools teach aspects of sexual education but this tends to have only a limited effect on the risk of unplanned pregnancy or of catching a sexually transmitted disease. Research shows that family values and parenting styles are the strongest protective factors against early sexual activity. Adolescents who have a close relationship with their parents in which they can talk maturely and openly about relationships and sex are less likely to seek advice from their same-aged peers or parts of the Internet that might not have been written by individuals with the self-esteem and health of younger people in mind. Social norms also have an effect – countries with older norms for when sexual activity is acceptable (and narrower types of situations where it would be acceptable, such as only during marriage) have average later age of first sexual experiences. Perhaps because males are permitted greater "sexual freedom" by many cultures, these age- and situation-related social norms for sex seem to have a greater influence in women than in men. But across all cultures and countries, many young people engage in sexual activities before the age at which society would view this as being acceptable. Interestingly, legal limits on the age at which sexual activity is permitted in different countries are only weakly related to the average age of actual first activity, or even to societal norms. Just because something is illegal, it does not always follow that everyone in a given society obeys the rule when it comes to sex.

Legal limits tend to be set in terms of arbitrary numbers, or whether a person of a given age would be able to legitimately "consent" to sex, i.e. be able to weigh up the benefits and risks, and arrive at a reasoned decision. On an individual level, what issues might be important in determining whether sex between two people is appropriate and "healthy"? Experts have suggested that both partners should willingly agree (i.e. sex is not forced, and it is consensual), that safe practices are used (e.g. using barrier contraception), that the act should not be done because of peer pressure or drugs (e.g. being intoxicated), and that the act should not be regretted afterwards. Using a scale that was developed to measure competence to make a decision about having sex based on the above principles, more than 70 percent of men and women who first had sex aged 13–14 years were probably not competent to do so at the time. That said, the study also found that around 30 percent of people who first had sex aged 18 years or above were also not competent.

Same-Gender Sexual Desire

Adolescence is a time when young people develop and to some extent craft their identities within society and among their peers, and part of this includes the establishment of sexual preferences. Sexual orientation is complicated and, contrary to classical beliefs, is not always static. It can fluctuate and change over time, especially in adolescence – a period when young people tend to experiment more. It relates not only to actual sexual practices but also to sexual fantasies, and to one's sense of identity. The precise effects of different processes (genetic, biological, psychological, and environmental) on the development of sexual orientation are controversial and have received relatively little scientific study due to this.

While sexual orientation is regarded by some as categorical (homosexual, heterosexual, or bisexual), others argue that it exists along a continuum. This continuous or scale-based approach suggests that sexual orientation exists somewhere between exclusive preference and sexual attraction toward the opposite sex, through to exclusive preference and sexual attraction toward the same sex. Societal attitudes toward homosexuality have been changing over time but still differ markedly depending on country, region, and economic development. Same-sex practices remain illegal in many parts of the world, and in some areas are even punishable by death. In Western societies, rapid changes have occurred to decriminalize same-sex activities and to protect people being discriminated against based on their sexual orientation, but in most cases these changes are relatively recent (the past 25–50 years).

What biological factors could be involved in sexual orientation? Twin studies have found that sexual orientation viewed in a binary way (heterosexuality or homosexuality) are moderately heritable (i.e. inherited), suggesting that genetic factors play a role. Chemical factors might also be at play. Homosexual men report an earlier average onset of puberty and an earlier age of first sexual experience, compared with heterosexual men. Some scientists speculate that this could be related to differences in the hormonal systems (e.g. testosterone), as these systems signal the onset of puberty, but direct evidence is lacking. Homosexual women do not report this difference in puberty onset or age of first sexual experience compared with heterosexual women. Homosexual men have, on average, a greater number of older brothers than heterosexual men. Homosexual men and women are statistically less likely to be right handed than their heterosexual counterparts. These differences are intriguing, but have not yet led to clear biological explanations. Attempts to explore biological associations with sexual orientation have often met with controversy, criticism, and even outright condemnation.

Biological mechanisms aside, homosexuality (or being in a minority group) raises vitally important unique health and well-being issues, which are considered further in Chapter 11.

Moving Beyond the Teenage Crush: Later Adolescence and Early Adulthood

Later in adolescence, Joanne would probably look humorously on the earlier crush on her history teacher, and would instead be exploring relationships with a greater focus on mutual and reciprocal interests. Humans are one of the few species with the capacity and predisposition to form romantic partnerships that are long term. Animals in nearly all other species meet, mate, and move on for more. There are notable exceptions to this, such as the prairie vole, which is mostly monogamous, staying with one partner for life, building a nest, and settling down with offspring – apart from occasionally mating with a random stranger (cheating). Penguins also tend to form pair bonds, but they do cheat a fair amount. This capacity to form long-term partnerships relates directly to the ability to form attachment bonds: a selective attachment that is enduring. Humans are especially prone to forming attachment bonds: we have exceptionally strong parent–child bonds and later romantic bonds, arising from (in part) biobehavioral synchrony, through which pairs of people (such as mother–child, partner–partner) develop similar hormone and physiological patterns over time: "Two hearts beat as one." One important hormone in romantic attachment bonds is oxytocin, the so-called "love hormone." Also important in being able to form sustained and more complicated relationships are the developmental improvements in our frontal lobes discussed earlier, which happen in late adolescence through to adulthood. The inferior frontal cortex and orbitofrontal cortex help stop us doing things that are not helpful for developing stable relationships, such as blurting out hurtful impulsive comments, or sleeping around with everyone in a nondirected way. The systems are not perfect!

Summary

We are born with desire: from birth, we crave mother's milk and form a close parental bond. Through evolution, nature has provided us with a common brain mechanism responsible for desire through regions including the ventral tegmentum and nucleus accumbens. It would not make sense in resource terms for the brain to develop completely different mechanisms for each possible desire we will experience through life, so there is a common mechanism or pathway. Without a desire mechanism, we would not eat, drink, exercise, form relationships, or reproduce. As we enter our teenage years, there are rapid changes in the circuit of desire and we experience sexual awakening in its broadest sense: priming for sex-relevant information in the environment, a fantasy sexual life, becoming fertile, and learning about our expressed sexuality and how this fits with our established position in society. There are further behavior and brain-remodeling changes as we move into adulthood, as we learn to form romantic bonds, rather than more egocentric attachments (the classical teenager crush) that might not be reciprocated or as long term. As providence gave us a mechanism for desire, so too do our brains have a mechanism for putting the brake on how we respond to it. Parts of the brain's frontal cortex develop to suppress our desires or put a cap on them – but these regions are not fully functional or optimal until our late 20s or even older.

Hence, the surge in desire at puberty and early adulthood can run unchecked, tempered only by parental input and cultural norms, which are thus exceptionally important during that time. This, along with the changes in our environmental setting (e.g. becoming more independent, moving away from parents, getting a job, or starting university), makes puberty and early adulthood a vulnerable time for developing out-of-control desires, or desires that lead to acts later regretted. Habits formed in this period set the scene for our adult existence, for better and for worse.

4   Healthy Sex

Lucy is 24 years old and works as a barista in a coffee shop chain. She has been in a relationship with her partner, Bob, for 7 years. Lucy's younger sister has just got married in a "shot-gun" wedding, after finding out she was pregnant with twins. Lucy, until now contented with her lot, suddenly worries whether she will pass the biological window and later regret not having children. Lucy also worries that she has lost interest in sex with Bob. She has been having a stressful time at work and after she gets home and eats the evening meal, she feels so tired that she needs to sleep. Bob confronted Lucy one evening: "You never want to be with me. Don't you like me anymore?" Since then, Bob has been sleeping in a separate bedroom. Lucy wonders if he masturbates when he is alone, preferring this to her own company. Lucy feels guilty that she hasn't had children and worries that sex isn't possible with Bob any more – she feels she must be the only person her age who has lost interest in sex but wants children.

Mr. and Mrs. Smith are an elderly couple who recently celebrated their 50th wedding anniversary. Both of the Smiths chose to move into a care home a few weeks ago because they were finding it difficult to cook and look after themselves due to health problems. When they moved into the nursing home, they were placed in separate bedrooms. John, the Manager of the care home, received a complaint from one of the nurses saying that she caught Mr. Smith engaging in sexual activity with Mrs. Smith after he sneaked into her room at night. John wonders whether is it normal for elderly people to have a sexual interest in each other.

Most of us spend very little time each day having sex, compared with other life activities such as going to work, eating, sleeping, or watching television. You have probably heard statistics in the media to the effect that men think about sex all the time or "once every 7 seconds." Measuring how often men and women think about sex each day is difficult because we might think about sex and not even consciously realize it. Also, how could researchers accurately record how often we think about sex, without making us think about sex more than normal? This is like the so-called "white elephant" phenomenon. Try this for a moment. If we tell you: "Don't think about a white elephant! Seriously, don't think about a white elephant, unless you normally think about a white elephant. We want you to press this counter and click it whenever you think about a white elephant." OK, did you click it? This is the same for measuring how often we think about sex. In asking people to record every perceived "sex" thought, this will automatically make us think about sex more. There are other factors that might influence the accuracy of recording how often people think about sex. Some people might be worried that the researcher would think they are abnormal if they acknowledge thinking about sex (to avoid this, many surveys are anonymous – but do people believe this?). Another issue is that we might not want to admit to ourselves that we think about sex all the time, or never.

These warnings aside, if studies are large enough, logically we should be able to approximate the "truth" about sex-related thoughts. One well-conducted study found that men thought about sex 19 times per day on average, while women thought about sex 10 times per day on average. How did this compare to other desire-related thoughts? In the same study, men thought about food on average 18 times per day, and women thought about food 15 times per day. This suggests that, in terms of our thought processes, we have sex thoughts to a similar extent as food thoughts. However, we spend about an hour a day eating but probably much less time than this engaging in sex per day if we take the average.

We do not have sex 10–19 times per day – every sex-related thought does not lead to an act. Why is this? This is partly because of our biological brake system (you just had a sex thought – whoops, it wouldn't be appropriate to make a move here in public). But also, having a thought does not mean there is an intention behind it – some thoughts are "null" or empty of meaning. You might have thought about the white elephants earlier, but that did not mean you wanted to go out and acquire a white elephant, or even look at white elephants on the Internet. Thoughts are not necessarily meaningful or significant behaviorally. In many forms of meditation, practitioners learn to recognize thoughts running through their minds and to accept them; people familiar with meditation learn that our minds can be full of random thoughts, many of which we would struggle to assign any meaning to, and we would certainly not act upon them. One interpretation for the lower frequency of sexual thoughts in women compared with men might be the idea that women on average are more focused on the emotional and bonding aspects of relationships but that men are more focused on the physicality of sex. In our first case example above, Lucy has temporarily lost interest in sex – probably because she is tired and stressed at work. Because her partner, Bob, has a lot of sexual thoughts, he feels extremely rejected when Lucy does not want to have sex. Being focused more on the physicality of sex, Bob assumes that Lucy does not have a sexual interest in him anymore, rather than thinking from her point of view. Rather than talking about the problem, they argue and start sleeping in separate bedrooms.

In this chapter, we want to cover several areas of healthy sexuality. Toward that end, we want first to examine topics that pertain largely to one's sexual feelings and thoughts, including masturbation and pornography, and then to focus on topics relevant to sexuality involving others, including duration/frequency of sex, how to increase interest in sex in couples, issues around infidelity, and sex in midlife and later life.

Masturbation

Masturbation refers to stimulation of the genitals to achieve pleasure, usually to the point of having an orgasm. Masturbation was a forbidden topic of discussion in many earlier societies – in fact, even now it is often not talked about very openly. Some traditional views held that masturbation was sinful because it involves obtaining pleasure without the intent of procreation (having children). This has perhaps fed forward into comments such as "If you touch yourself, you'll go blind" to dissuade adolescent boys from masturbating. There is no convincing scientific evidence that masturbating has negative health consequences. Masturbation is only a problem if it causes distress to the person (if it gets out of control or too frequent), or interferes with life or relationships (e.g. excessive masturbation so that we do not go to work, or cannot have sex with a partner because we overdid it). Masturbation can also be problematic if it breaches social norms or legal rules (e.g. if an individual masturbates in public).

The National Survey of Sexual Health and Behavior, conducted at Indiana University in the USA, assessed sexual practices in over 5,000 people across a broad age range. In people aged 18–19 years, 81 percent of men and 60 percent of women had masturbated in the past year. Similar results were reported in middle age, so this is not just a phenomenon in teenagers! The oldest group considered were aged 70 or more – 46 percent of men and 33 percent of women in this group had masturbated in the past year. So there seems to be some reduction in masturbation as we age but not by much. Masturbating with one's partner was also fairly common: around 40 percent of people (men and women) reported masturbating with a partner (or masturbating one's partner) in the past year, but this rate reduced considerably in older age. The survey also examined younger people: 62 percent of boys and 40 percent of girls aged 14–15 years reported masturbating alone during the past year, whereas sexual acts with others were relatively uncommon in this age group. Based on this, masturbation can be viewed as a normal part of sexuality in men and women from adolescence through to older age. Do younger people masturbate? Even children can sometimes become aroused in terms of their genitalia; some children then "fiddle" as this is self-soothing, but this probably is not triggered by sex-related thoughts or drives until close to puberty.

In terms of how frequently people should masturbate, there is considerable variation in how much people masturbate, and it fluctuates throughout our lives due to things like health, stress, work and home schedules, desire, and dynamics in a partnership. Assuming it is not interfering with your life in some fashion, there is no "normal" amount of masturbation, and masturbation is not harmful, even if you do it often.

Health Benefits of Masturbation

The positive effects of masturbation have not been studied much – this probably reflects the fact that masturbation is still considered taboo or somehow immoral in some places. Why would government and charitable bodies fund research on this topic? They would be criticized. In our clinical experience, masturbation can have positive consequences for people – men and women we see clinically report that it can relieve tension and anxiety, aid sleep, improve mood, and increase energy, and mutual masturbation can increase emotional closeness in couples. If couples are worried about sexually transmitted diseases, masturbation can constitute a relatively low-risk activity compared with oral sex or sexual intercourse. For couples wishing to avoid pregnancy, mutual masturbation is an alternative to sexual intercourse with a very low pregnancy risk (there is a theoretical but low risk of pregnancy if semen is spread from male to female genitalia due to lack of caution).

One idea that you may have come across in health magazines is that male masturbation might reduce the risk of prostate cancer. The prostate gland is walnut sized and sits at the base of the bladder in men; it produces fluid that, along with sperm, is released when men ejaculate. Prostate cancer is one of the most common types of cancer in men. An Australian study asked approximately 1,000 men with prostate cancer and 1,000 men without prostate cancer about their sexual histories. The researchers found that the more ejaculations men had over time, the lower the later risk of prostate cancer. The effect seemed especially strong for the number of ejaculations when men were in their 20s. The number of sexual partners did not correlate with the risk of prostate cancer in this study. These findings suggest that masturbation might be protective against prostate cancer. There are several possible explanations behind this finding, such as that regular masturbation could reduce levels of hormones or help to prevent accumulation of prostate fluid that has cancer risk. Since that study, very large-scale datasets have been developed (including from studies following people up over time) supporting the link between more frequent ejaculation and lower later risk of prostate cancer.

Another intriguing area of research is in Catholic priests, who generally abstain from all forms of sexual practice (including masturbation). In one research study, information about more than 1,000 Catholic priests was collected. The researchers examined whether the rate of deaths from different causes, including from prostate cancer, was higher or lower in the priests compared with the background population. They found that the priests were approximately 50 percent more likely to have died from prostate cancer than expected, but they were much less likely to have died from lung cancer than expected. Another study in 6,000 Catholic priests found that they had lower than expected rates of multiple types of cancer, including lower rates of prostate cancer. It is hard to conclude much from this because the two studies had conflicting results and Catholic priests are likely to differ from the background population in many ways, such as in the types and volumes of food consumed, other desire-related behaviors besides sex, their degree of human contact, and so on.

Thus, regular masturbation might reduce the risk of later prostate cancer in men. But for both men and women, most experts agree that masturbation is a normal part of our sexual repertoire and should not be seen as shameful or abnormal.

Masturbation in Relationships

If one person masturbates separately from their partner, does this have a negative effect on the relationship? If a man catches his wife masturbating in the shower, or vice versa, should they be upset, or just carry on and ignore what they saw, or should they mention it but jovially? You might be surprised to hear that in large anonymous surveys, the majority of married men and women reported that they masturbate separately from their partner at times. In fact, masturbation may help a relationship. Self-pleasure offers an opportunity to explore what turns you on and gives you pleasure, which can help you communicate your sexual desires to your partner. One study found that married women who masturbated had more orgasms and sexual desire, that it boosted self-esteem, and, overall, resulted in greater satisfaction in marriage and sex. In terms of the relationship, many therapists would agree that couples should discuss masturbation. Couples should openly discuss the comfort level of solo sex with each other.

Most couples, at some point in the relationship, have a gap in sexual interest – typically one partner has more interest in sex than the other. Rather than harassing the less interested partner for more sex, masturbation might be a way, for some, of avoiding the issue and "balancing out" the differences in sex drive. Masturbation could also be a way of fulfilling sex cravings if a partner is not available – while traveling, or due to health conditions. Early work by the Kinsey Institute for Research in Sex, Gender, and Reproduction at Indiana University found that women who had masturbated before marriage were more likely to achieve orgasm with their partner during marriage. Since then, more recent research has found that married women who masturbated had higher levels of marital satisfaction. On discovering our nearest and dearest masturbating alone, it is tempting to feel hurt – does this mean our partner is not interested in us? The evidence does not generally suggest this to be the case. Self-masturbation is about quick pleasure rather than intimacy with another; it is a private rather than an intimate act, serving a biological rather than a higher-level psychological need. On average, college students who masturbated more frequently were found to have sex more frequently. Masturbation might serve to maintain or promote interest in sex with our partner, by keeping the "system in shape," which can add to closeness rather than being a negative habit.

There are situations in which self-masturbation can be unhealthy for a relationship. Too much self-masturbation can lead to a narrowing of sexual interests, so that a person may lose interest in couple-centered sexual activities, or want to engage in mutual sex activities but find this physically difficult as they are "sexed out." In these cases, we recommend that couples talk about it openly and consider couples counseling, because it would suggest that it is a problem.

Pornography

When one thinks of masturbation, the topic naturally turns toward pornography. Although clearly masturbation can involve sexual fantasies of one's own making, pornography generally is used for purposes of masturbation. Pornography has a long and colorful history (even the definition is questionable; we generally are referring to any materials intended to arouse erotic feelings). Vast quantities of depictions of sexual acts (both heterosexual and homosexual) have been recovered from Ancient Greek and Roman civilizations. The *Kama Sutra*, an ancient Hindu text from around the second century CE, was written as a guide to good living, encapsulating prose and poems. It includes practical advice relating to 64 types of sex acts, and is a top seller in online book sales in the present day.

In modern times, there were extensive prohibitions on pornographic material even in Western countries until relatively recently, while pornography remains prohibited in other parts of the world. It was possible in the past to restrict access to pornography by having laws about printing pornography and distributing it. But now, free pornography is readily accessible by virtually everyone who has access to the Internet, although attempts are made to prevent children being exposed to pornography by using website "blocking software." As with other topics to do with sexuality, pornography use is not discussed openly very often. Teenagers might talk about and share pornography with each other, of course not telling their parents. Adults, including parents, might look at pornography (including during sex together) but never tell anyone, especially their teenaged children. If we asked whether you use pornography, and you do, would you answer truthfully? If not, why not? The topic is private and out of bounds because it is taboo, and there is a sense that pornography viewing might be wrong or, at the least, embarrassing. Having said that, recent data showed that daily visits to Pornhub, a popular online pornography site (of which there are over 4 million sites), exceeded 100 million. So, even if no one talks about pornography, clearly many people are consuming it.

One objection to viewing pornography is that it may involve exploitation of men and women who make the pornographic material (the actors). So, by acquiring and viewing these types of material, we might be encouraging exploitation, or indirectly exposing the actors to other risks (e.g. sexually transmitted diseases). The corollary to this argument is that, if pornography actors ("porn stars") make material without coercion and are fully aware of the benefits and risks, and consent to their involvement in making pornography, can it truly be said that they are being exploited? We do not pass judgment one way or the other as this is a complex area for which individuals can hold very different viewpoints. There are types of pornography for which there would be virtually universal consensus that they should be prohibited – such as pornography involving minors, exploitation, or coercion.

Questions of acceptability and morality aside, how common is mainstream pornography use? In a Danish study, a representative sample of 700 adults aged 18–30 years (men and women, average age 25 years) was asked to complete a questionnaire about pornography use and related behaviors. Overall, 98 percent of the men and 80 percent of the women admitted to viewing pornography at some point in their lives, while 63 percent of men and 14 percent of women reported viewing pornography in the past week. The most common context for using pornography was when alone in men, and when with a partner in women, and the average amount of time spent viewing pornography in each week was 80 minutes in men and 20 minutes in women. The strongest predictors of higher pornography use were being male, being younger, having an earlier age when first viewing pornography, and greater frequency of masturbation. What can we conclude from this? Denmark has a liberal outlook – it was the first country in the world to legalize pornography (pornographic texts were made legal in 1967 and pornographic imagery was made legal in 1969). These statistics suggest that in more liberal parts of the world, pornography use is common and is closely linked with masturbation and partaking in sex acts with others. Of course, it is harder to study pornography use in parts of the world where it is more taboo, or even forbidden, but available data indicate that pornography use is not uncommon even in cultures that ban it.

Duration of Sex

To be a "sensitive lover," and if you believe the television, we should all be spending hours having sexual intercourse each time. In order to measure the length of time spent on sex per intercourse, we need to define it. Sex could include the flirting, foreplay, and sex itself, through to orgasm/completion, but most research focuses on the time between first penile insertion and the man's ejaculation for simplicity of measurement. When researchers asked 500 couples to record length of sex using stopwatches and this definition, they found that the length of sexual intercourse varied considerably. The average amount of time for sexual intercourse (penile insertion to ejaculation) was 5.5 minutes – this contrasts significantly with what many might expect based on media portrayals or literature! The quickest sexual intercourse was apparently 33 seconds and the slowest was 44 minutes. The average length of time for sexual intercourse was similar across countries, even when comparing what would be considered conservative countries versus countries with more liberal/less strict sexual attitudes. The research found that older people tended to have quicker sexual intercourse, which might run against the idea of slower or longer sexual intercourse being indicative of closer relationships, or more loving relationships.

Frequency of Sex

In single people, and in couples, there are vast differences in how much sex people partake in. This can also change over time – there can even be long periods of time when we do not feel like sex because we lack a partner, just have no interest, or are interested but busy pursuing other areas of life. Loss of interest in sex can be normal but can also – for some – suggest psychological difficulties, interpersonal problems, or physical health problems for which there can be a role for support and treatment (discussed in Chapters 5 and 7, respectively). Interest in sex can vary because of medications, having children at home, substance use, recent bereavements, stress in general, problems in the relationship, or a multitude of other issues. Not having much interest in sex in a relationship does not always mean there is a problem with the relationship.

As with our earlier discussion about the average amount of time taken for sexual intercourse, the average number of times people have sex per time period (such as per week, month, or year) varies considerably. On average, young adult couples have sex one to two times per week, while older couples in longer-term relationships have sex on average one to two times per month. About 20 percent of long-term couples have sex only occasionally (less than once per month) or even never. Research shows that if both people in the partnership are comfortable with limited or no sex, they can be otherwise contented in the partnership, because they might assign more importance to other joint activities that they consider more essential. In a large study in the UK, fewer than half of the people surveyed said they felt satisfied with their sex lives, but most people did not rank their sex lives as being in the top three most important factors in their relationships. People tended to rank honesty and good communication higher. Most people ranked their relationships as being good despite not having complete satisfaction with their sex lives. So being completely satisfied with sex is not the norm, and is not a requirement for having a meaningful and contented relationship.

Increasing Sexual Interest in a Relationship

Lack of sex in a relationship is not always a problem. Difficulties arise when a couple have different sex drives, or different expectations about sex. For example, one member of a couple could lose interest in sex because they are stressed at work and not sleeping well, while the other member of a couple might wonder if the person no longer finds them sexually attractive. Couples may have different attitudes toward sex, and these issues cannot be explored and resolved if they do not talk about sex. If there is an issue, it is better to discuss it openly in a fresh frame of mind when not tired, and to avoid losing one's temper. There are countless self-help books devoted to sex tips for couples. Here we suggest some tips or pointers that couples can find useful. If one person feels "pressured" to have sex, this can be a real mood killer. If this happens, it can be helpful for the other person to take the pressure off – to show emotional warmth and engage in joint activities (surprise dates, or going on a walk together) without any expectation of sex for at least a few weeks. Another good idea is to change the setting: people can get stuck in a loop of going to work, cooking, eating, going to work, cooking, eating, and so on. Try going on holiday together or even just doing something more straightforward to break the routine. Time apart is not always a bad thing – it can be used for reflection, and might help a couple to better appreciate what they get from a relationship, rather than just the problems.

In our experience, couples can be reluctant to go for therapy – confidential therapy for couples is available in many countries and regions. We advise people to have couples therapy even if they feel their relationship is healthy and free from problems. Being in a long-term relationship results in a steep learning curve for many and is a commitment; engaging in couples therapy can be a clear sign that a couple wants to make their relationship as strong as possible, and is a positive thing, independent of not having major issues in the relationship. Last but by no means least, if one person in a couple has noticed a drop in their libido (or, alternatively, excessive sex drive) that does not have a clear cause, it can be helpful to discuss this with a family doctor to help rule out medical causes. Medical causes of sexual difficulties are discussed in Chapter 7.

Infidelity

Not surprisingly, few scientists have chosen to specialize in the research area of infidelity! There have been surveys that asked people about infidelity but little controlled research. The problem with surveys about cheating is that: most of them have been done by magazines or newspapers so the findings could be biased; we do not know if those people who completed the surveys were representative of the general population; and we do not know that there is even a common definition for "cheating." In a survey of 2,500 men via an online fitness magazine, 58 percent said they had cheated on a partner at least once, most often with a close friend or work colleague. Of men who said they had never cheated, around a third said that they might cheat if they thought they could get away with it. The charity Relate, which runs relationship counseling in the UK, conducted a representative survey of over 6,000 men and women. Nearly a quarter of people surveyed admitted to physically cheating on their partner at least once (now or in the past), while 41 percent of women and 35 percent of men reported that a partner had cheated on them. Individuals with a disability or long-term health problems had a higher chance of being cheated on, which might suggest an increased risk of cheating if a partner is unwell and less sexually active. Overall, 33 percent of people said that they checked their partner's telephone or otherwise checked up on them to see if they had been cheating.

The available peer-reviewed research studies (i.e. those that go through processes to help assure quality and interpretation of results) suggest that in a long-term relationship, the average chance of a partner cheating at some point is 15–25 percent. The General Social Survey conducted annually by the University of Chicago using a representative national sample about infidelity have found fairly consistent results over the years – that is, every year, approximately 10 percent of spouses admit cheating (12 percent of men 7 percent of women).

The risk of cheating is lower in relationships in which partners have more similar sex drive and fewer unresolved problems or arguments. Higher spirituality also seems to be protective. Discovery of cheating is one of the biggest triggers for relationships breaking down, and also for people starting relationship counseling to try to fix things.

What can we learn from the statistics? If there are problems in a relationship, including things like one partner struggling because the other person's sex drive is very different, it is better to address these earlier on rather than to push the issues to one side and ignore them.

Midlife Crisis

The phrase "midlife crisis" refers to issues of identity and self-confidence that can happen in middle age. The stereotypical television idea of a midlife crisis would be a man in his 50s who buys an expensive sports car, suddenly takes up interests more suited to a 20-year-old, and believes he is living the playboy lifestyle. Having a midlife crisis might seem to be a trite term, but is there evidence that a midlife crisis is a true phenomenon with a medical basis?

Some scientists think a midlife crisis is a real thing, but others dispute it. When researchers questioned individuals in several different countries, they identified an "inverted U" model for human happiness. What they mean by "inverted U" is that if we draw a graph plotting age (from 20 years through to 70 years) against overall life satisfaction, we start with high life satisfaction in youth, then things increasingly dip to reach a low point in our 40s to 50s, and then they increase again, with higher satisfaction as we get older. What we call a midlife crisis could just be getting over this dip in life satisfaction – we might suddenly seem invigorated with a lust for life once again. Viewed this way, a midlife crisis might refer to different ways we change as we get over this low point. This middle-aged dip and later surge in life satisfaction happens in both men and women. There are also some medical explanations that might account for a midlife crisis.

During the menopause, which typically happens in middle age (48–55 years), women experience a profound drop in the levels of estrogen in their body, and the ovaries stop producing eggs. This affects people differently, but common symptoms include mood swings, loss of libido, physical symptoms (sweating, flushes, racing heart, headaches, vaginal dryness/soreness), and trouble sleeping. Because this biological process is likely to coincide with the "dip" in life satisfaction described above, this might make for a "double whammy." The body usually adapts gradually to the menopause, so that these symptoms settle down after a few years. These processes could contribute to a midlife crisis for some.

Men in middle age experience gradual decline in levels of certain hormones including testosterone, and some men are affected more than others. When men have low testosterone on blood tests and associated symptoms, some doctors refer to this as "andropause." Symptoms can include loss of libido, mood swings, fatigue, and difficulties getting an erection (erectile dysfunction).

Sex in Later Life

In our second vignette at the top of this chapter, we discussed a married couple, Mr. and Mrs. Smith, who moved into a nursing home. The care staff made the assumption that Mr. and Mrs. Smith would not be sexually active with each other because of their age. Mr. Smith is caught in a compromising position with Mrs. Smith in her bedroom one night. It is completely normal for older people to engage in sex-related activities including sexual intercourse. Many studies have shown that older people continue to desire sexual intimacy and to engage in sexual activities. This is quite different from what wider society might assume to be the case.

When a group of older women with partners were asked about their sexuality in Australia, very diverse attitudes were found – some people had stopped all sex, while others were currently having more sex than they did when they were younger (including masturbation). A common issue raised by the participants in the study was that they still had sexual interests but were constrained in the frequency or nature of sex acts because of medications reducing their sexual performance, or because of physical health difficulties. Healthcare professionals seemed reluctant to discuss sexual health problems with these older people – more so than when they were younger. It is important not to assume that older people are no longer sexually active.

Summary

In adulthood, our desires, including sexual desire, are not static. In this chapter, we have seen that sexual practices and relationships in adulthood can be extremely diverse, without being necessarily abnormal or problematic. Traditional views that some sex-related behaviors are rare or abnormal do not match up with modern existence – self-masturbation and pornography use are extremely common, including in long-term relationships. Older people can have a higher sex drive than their younger counterparts. Appreciating when sexual practices are normal, or when they are going out of kilter and might need external support or help to manage, can be challenging, especially for couples, because relationships involve many assumptions about the other partner that can be different from the reality. For these reasons, we recommend couples counseling in general, rather than only for couples who feel they have specific relationship problems.

5 Too Little Sex

Theresa is a 57-year-old woman who has been married for 30 years and has had three children during that time. During her marriage, Theresa has generally enjoyed her sexual relationship with her husband, and both she and her husband have felt fulfilled by it. Over the past few years, however, Theresa has noticed that she feels much less interested in sex than she had previously. Initially, Theresa had not noticed the change, and felt that she and her husband had sex as often as they needed to, and that he felt the same way. After a while, however, her husband started commenting that he felt disappointed that they did not have sex more often. Theresa thought it was just a short-lived issue but then noticed that the lack of sexual intimacy had persisted over a longer period of time. This decrease in amount of sex did not bother Theresa directly, but her husband seemed to be getting increasingly frustrated, leading to strain and conflict within the marriage. Despite having less interest in sex, Theresa still feels that she loves her husband and wants to keep their relationship going and ensure it is healthy. Theresa feels stuck and is unsure how to make things work, or even what has caused her to lose so much of her interest in having sex in the first place. She would love to find a treatment for her reduced interest but does not know what to do in order to fix what she sees as the central problem that is undermining the stability of her relationship. Without something to fix her situation with her husband, she worries that this change in sexual desire could mean the end of her marriage.

Stewart is a 21-year-old male in college. Stewart recently started dating a new woman and is excited about the relationship. Stewart and his partner typically have intercourse one or two times per week, and both of them enjoy the sex. Recently, however, Stewart's girlfriend has been complaining that the two do not have sex as often as they should, and has been asking if it is because Stewart is not attracted to her anymore. Stewart, in contrast, thought that they were having plenty of sex, and was surprised when his partner suggested otherwise. Since then, Stewart has been extremely worried that something is wrong with him as he does not want to have sex with his girlfriend more frequently. He has tried to force himself to have sex more frequently but feels as though he cannot get aroused that often. Eventually, Stewart sought out several different aphrodisiacs online and has been trying different options over a series of weeks. Unfortunately, none of the herbs, supplements, or compounds he has tried has resulted in any increase in his sexual desire. Stewart feels like a failure and is concerned that something is wrong with his brain, his hormones, or even his genitals. He has no idea whom to ask about his situation, and feels too embarrassed to talk to his partner about it. Stewart is concerned that his partner is going to leave him if he does not find a way to fix his problem as soon as possible.

Sexual desire is something frequently described in terms of having "too much" or "too little" of it, and what regular people can do to increase or decrease that level. Often omitted in those conversations, however, is a discussion of what typical desire is, the factors that can give rise to heightened or lowered sexual desire, and if there truly is a problem with a given level of sexual desire for an individual person. This chapter, and the one following, explore these ideas of low and high desire, and discuss what these levels are, what can cause them, why they can be important, and (when necessary) what options are possible to treat them.

Levels of Sexual Desire

When discussing the idea of sexual desire and the level of that desire, one of the fundamental things that should be addressed is how much desire is normal and healthy. Although many resources are eager to point out how they have the perfect tips to bolster a lack-luster libido, little is offered to explain what the boost to "normalcy" would look like. The reason for this could be that there is no true "normal" level of sexual desire, and it is something that is relative to the exemplars we compare ourselves with, whether realistic or not. Levels of desire – in terms of both wanting sex and getting aroused – can shift over the years, or from week to week or partner to partner. Thus, one is left with the unsatisfying (although possibly accurate) message that "normal" levels of sexual desire are a moving target that we can never truly meet. There is no right or normal amount of sexual desire, just what is right for the person.

Given this, it may be necessary to shift the manner in which we conceptualize "amounts" of sexual desire and what is normal/healthy. Rather than attempting to establish the ideal standard for the quantity and magnitude of sexual desire, desire can be seen as existing along a continuum, ranging from individuals with very high levels to those who have almost no sexual desire. Everyone exists on this spectrum; some will be higher, some lower, but all fall along the continuum based on individual preference and proclivities. In this depiction, there is no set value for a "normal" amount of sexual desire that we should all be hoping to achieve. Instead, it is possible to recognize the importance of individual variation, and individual variation over time, and that these variations are inherently neither good nor bad, just as the degree to which a person enjoys action movies or playing sports is neither a good nor a bad thing. The level of sexual desire can be seen simply as a characteristic of the person, which may or may not align with sexual and romantic partners.

This take on sexual desire, while a potential shift from previous conceptualizations, may not lessen the strain that people such as Stewart and Theresa experience when they feel that their level of sexual desire is falling short of what their partners expect or what they themselves feel that it "should be" – at least, it may not seem to accomplish this on its most basic level. What this perspective shift does offer, however, is to normalize sexual behavior and desire across a far wider spectrum of levels. Rather than "fixing" Stewart's lower level of desire relative to his girlfriend, it is possible instead to describe it as just that: lower relative to her but potentially normal and healthy by Stewart's own standards. Thus, although conceptualizing a healthy level of sexual desire as existing along a wider spectrum may not in itself resolve points of conflict, it does provide a starting point for a wider discussion of low, high, and "normal" levels of sexual desire. While this may seem abstract, the take-away message can be boiled down to the simple idea that if you are comfortable and happy with your baseline level of sexual desire after eliminating the pressure that comes from cultural norms, partners and other outside sources, then it is likely a healthy and normal level for you.

Low Desire and Hypoactive Sexual Desire Disorder

Even after recognizing the spectrum of healthy levels of sexual desire that are possible, a number of people fall outside that range and experience levels of sexual desire that are notably low to the point that they cause the individual significant distress or additional difficulty. When the level of desire reaches a clinically low level, this is called hypoactive sexual desire disorder (HSDD). HSDD can affect both men and women. Discussions regarding HSDD have often focused on women, but problems with low desire can be a factor for either gender, although causal factors and presentations may differ in some regards, based on biological, sociocultural, and individual factors.

The presentation of HSDD may differ between men and women slightly, but the diagnosis can be formally made when the person reports persistently or recurrently deficient (or absent) sexual/erotic thoughts or fantasies and desire for sexual activity. This may show itself in several ways: little or no interest in sexual activity, no or few sexual thoughts, no or few attempts to initiate sexual activity or respond to a partner's initiation, no or little sexual pleasure/excitement in the vast majority (75–100 percent) of sexual experiences, no or little sexual interest in internal or external erotic stimuli, and no or few genital/nongenital sensations in the vast majority (75–100 percent) of sexual experiences. For the diagnosis of HSDD, symptoms must persist for at least 6 months. Simply having lower desire than one's partner is not sufficient for a diagnosis.

Data suggest that 34 percent of women between the ages of 18 and 74 experience decreased sexual interest often or most of the time. When pursued by their partner or potential partner, however, women explained that they experienced arousal and interest in sexual activity. Thus, some women might not experience much sexual desire until appropriate stimulation occurs. In contrast, an estimated 15 percent of the general male population experience HSDD.

While an individual must meet certain criteria to receive a formal diagnosis of HSDD, low sexual desire can be a significant problem, even when it does not meet the criteria for HSDD. Given this, the present chapter will discuss problematic low sexual desire in a more inclusive sense, rather than distinguishing between HSDD and more general problematic low sexual desire.

Physical and Medical Causes of Low Sexual Desire

Many people struggling with low sexual desire feel that their problem is due to a personal failing and that they should be able to just "snap out of it," but it is important to bear in mind that there are a number of medical and biological factors that can give rise to diminished sexual desire. Dysregulation in systems related to hormones and neuro-transmitters, chronic diseases such as diabetes and hypothyroidism, physical injuries, and psychological problems such as depression can all have unwanted negative effects on the level of sexual desire. Some of these factors are unique to men or women, but many show notable impact regardless of sex.

Medical Conditions

Several medical conditions may result in low sexual desire. If any are suspected, a person should consult their primary doctor for a thorough physical examination and possibly blood tests. Treatments for these medical conditions may result in improved sexual drive.

Hypogonadism

Hypogonadism refers to diminished functional activity of the gonads (i.e. the testes in males and ovaries in females). This condition results in decreased production of sex hormones and therefore people have low testosterone levels or low estradiol hormone levels.

Hypertension

Hypertension, also known as high blood pressure, is a long-term medical condition in which the blood pressure in the arteries is persistently elevated. Particularly in men, this condition can result in reduced sexual interest. High blood pressure can damage the lining of blood vessels and causes arteries to harden and narrow, resulting in limited blood flow. This means less blood is able to flow to the penis. For some men, the decreased blood flow makes it difficult to achieve and maintain erections. High blood pressure can also interfere with ejaculation. Taken together, these can result in reduced sexual desire.

Hypothyroidism

This a common disorder in which the thyroid gland does not produce enough thyroid hormone. This can cause a number of symptoms, such as poor ability to tolerate cold, a feeling of tiredness, constipation, depression, and weight gain. Hypothyroidism results in a slowed metabolism, and this in turn may cause other organs and glands to slow down, such as the reproductive organs and the adrenal glands, which produce hormones that are converted into sex hormones (testosterone, estrogen, and progesterone). Low levels of these hormones may in turn result in a low sex drive.

Obesity

Obesity is defined by a body mass index (BMI) of 30 or higher. BMI uses a simple calculation based on the ratio of someone's height and weight squared (BMI = kg divided by m^2). Decades of research have shown that BMI provides a good estimate of "fatness" and also correlates well with important health outcomes such as heart disease, diabetes, cancer, and overall mortality. Very obese people are 25 times more likely to report problems in their sex lives compared with normal-weight people. Fat tissues contain enzymes, and one prevalent enzyme called aromatase converts testosterone into estradiol. When fat tissues increase, so do the concentrations of aromatase, which then starts breaking down testosterone. This leads to a lower sex drive.

Depressed Mood

A depressed mood is characterized by sadness, loss of interest, and lack of motivation. A symptom of depression is a lack of interest in sex and a low libido. It may be due to low levels of sex hormones as both testosterone (in men) or estrogen/progesterone (in women) have been able to improve mood and sexual desire in some people. Antidepressants may also play a role as they often improve mood and perhaps indirectly improve sexual desire. At the same time, many antidepressants can have the opposite effect of reducing sexual desire or otherwise interfering with sexual function, and doctors often fail to ask about this potential side effect.

Anxiety

Anxiety results in excessive worry and concern over life events such as finances, health, or future plans. Anxiety often produces a lack of or decreased sexual desire. The exact biological reason for this remains unclear. Anxiety distracts a person, and when we have problems focusing and concentrating, we often have lower sexual drive (remember, sexual desire is as much a mental exercise as a physical drive). Anxiety can also map onto worries about sexual performance, which feed into a cycle where worries lead to sex problems, which then reinforce the worries. Treatment for anxiety often improves sexual desire.

Alcohol Use

The use of alcohol reduces both men's and women's sexual sensitivity. In addition, in men, alcohol can cause difficulties getting and maintaining an erection, while women may experience reduced lubrication, find it harder to have an orgasm, or may have orgasms that are less intense. Many people mistakenly believe that alcohol is an aphrodisiac. On the one hand, alcohol can impair our "behavioral brain brake" leading to sex behaviors that we might not otherwise do, but on the other hand, over time, too much alcohol can actually reduce or eliminate sexual drive.

Medications

Medications such as certain antidepressants (selective serotonin reuptake inhibitors, which raise serotonin levels), opioid pain medications (which can lower testosterone and affect libido) and possibly oral contraceptives can lower levels of sex hormones, including testosterone, and therefore may negatively affect libido.

While the previously noted conditions and situations may have hormonal or specific biological associations that may give rise to lower levels of sexual desire, many severe and/or persistent health conditions can impact sexual desire indirectly. Significant impairment of mobility, overall energy, or other factors may limit interest in sex simply due to an individual's perceived ability to have "good" sex, or any sex at all. For many people, these types of impairment have no less of an impact on their sexual desire, even if they lack a specific direct connection to desire. As will be discussed in later sections, perceived ability to have sex, concerns about sexual performance, and a myriad of other psychological factors can also give rise to lower levels of sexual desire.

A Specific Note on Hormones

In the case of men with low sexual desire, research to date has suggested that androgens, with particular emphasis on testosterone, play a notable role in sexual desire, whereas the link in women is less clear. Although testosterone is typically associated with the development of masculine characteristics, previous research on sexual desire has suggested that testosterone is related to both sexual desire and the drive to initiate sexual activity, which would indicate that some amount of testosterone is necessary to experience sexual desire. For men who are unable to produce sufficient testosterone due to conditions such as hypogonadism, low sexual desire is relatively common. In these cases, low levels of testosterone can be associated with dysfunction in several areas, including erectile dysfunction, diminished desire, and difficulty achieving orgasm. Levels of testosterone beyond typical levels are not, however, associated with additional increases in sexual desire, contrary to common assumptions. Thus, many of the over-the-counter testosterone or testosterone-like products that advertise increased male sexual potency may be either useless or unnecessary, particularly if a man's testosterone level is already within normal parameters. Other hormones may also play a notable role in male sexual desire, but androgens have been the primary focus of existing literature.

Hormones likely play a similarly important role in women. While androgens are most commonly associated with men, they may also play some role in establishing and maintaining sexual desire in women. Although the role of testosterone in women differs from its role in men, it is notable that women with female androgen deficiency syndrome, which is associated with low circulating levels of testosterone, report lower sexual desire, receptivity, and pleasure relative to women without the condition. Results from additional studies assessing possible relationships between testosterone and sexual desire in women have been inconsistent, however, with different studies reporting varying associations (or lack thereof) between androgens and sexual desire in women. The lack of consensus on how testosterone and other androgens impact female desire makes it a relatively hazy target for medical assessment when attempting to treat low sexual desire. The impact of varying ratios of androgens and other sex hormones, cyclic variations in hormone levels, and other contributing factors limit the potential clinical utility of hormonal assessments for most women struggling with low sexual desire. For those with a predisposing condition such as female androgen deficiency syndrome, however, hormonal assessments with an endocrinologist may be beneficial due to the increased risk of dysregulation from a pre-existing condition. When considering women with low sexual desire as a whole, the possible cause of the low desire is likely to be too variable to be consistently associated with a specific hormonal dysregulation.

Interestingly, treatment studies assessing estrogen, androgens, and combined androgen–estrogen treatment options for HSDD found that the combined androgen–estrogen treatment showed the greatest improvement in symptoms. There are, however, only limited findings on the safety of long-term use of testosterone supplements in women for the purposes of treating low sexual desire. Given this, most women should address other possible causes for low sexual desire before assessing hormonal levels as a possible cause of low sexual desire.

While androgens often receive the most attention when assessing sexual desire, other hormones have also been suggested as possible factors in initiating, maintaining, or stopping sexual desire, particularly in women. It should be noted, however, that these hormones likely play a role in sexual behavior and desire in both men and women, despite the fact that the majority of research on these hormones and their role in sexual behavior and desire has been conducted in women. Estrogen potentially facilitates permissive feelings toward sexual desire. Progesterone potentially modulates receptivity relating to sex and sexual desire. Prolactin appears to inhibit sexual excitement and could thus indirectly impair sexual desire. Oxytocin may help facilitate orgasms. If orgasms are impaired, individuals may feel less motivated or interested in sex without the reward of an orgasm.

Levels of Sexual Desire Fluctuate

Sexual desire is not static – people can have fluctuating levels of desire throughout their lives. This makes evolutionary sense. Our brains are probably not wired to think of sex when a saber-toothed tiger is attacking. Sexual drive is typically greatest when stress or anxiety is less. Therefore, when we are working on our careers, we often think less about sex than after we have attained our goals and have free time. Relatedly, stress in our lives will make our sexual drive less in many cases, and this may be family stress, health issues, or financial stress. Some people may engage more in sex during stress, but it is not always clear whether this is due to increased desire or simply a means of avoidance and distraction. Other external events can also affect desire such as meeting someone new and exciting versus being with the same person and having the same sexual routine for many years. One expects the former to heighten our sexual drive while the latter can contribute to lower sexual drive.

Body Image and Sexual Desire

Body image contributes to low sexual drive. Most people dislike some aspect of their appearance, but when body image concerns are more pronounced, it is common for the person to have less interest in sexual activity. This may be due to embarrassment from someone seeing them naked, or from poor self-esteem about some part of their body or lack of control over weight. Body image may be a problem for both men and women and is often difficult for someone to admit to their sexual partner. They may avoid or minimize sexual contact, and this can lead the other person ironically to believe they are not attractive. Of course, the relationship we have with our bodies and our sexual drive is complicated. Although poor body self-esteem lowers our interest in sex, studies have also shown that 35–40 percent of both men and women report that unpleasant sexual experiences cause negative feelings about their bodies. Thus, although the directionality of the influences of body image and sexual drive may be unclear, it is safe to say that the way we see our bodies is linked to our interest in sex. Ultimately, when people feel that a relationship is safe and trusting, they should discuss these concerns. There are also successful professional talk therapies that focus on improving body image.

The Role of Our Partner

Given the above issues, there may be multiple reasons for low sexual drive in any individual. For those in relationships, however, issues of the partner or of the relationship may contribute to the low sex drive. Alternatively, of course, the low sex drive of one person may create issues within the partnership and in the unaffected partner. One can therefore assume that, given these complex issues surrounding sex, there has been considerable attention focused on the problems of low or no sex partnerships. In these relationships, usually one partner has a very low libido or there is a significant discrepancy in sexual desire between the couple. The longer couples avoid sexual contact, the harder it becomes to break the cycle, and the longer they refrain from sexual contact, the more they tend to blame each other.

Reasons for low sexual drive by one partner can be anywhere from simple to complex. The other person may not be attentive sexually any longer, the sexual experience may have become commonplace or boring, or one person feels taken for granted (e.g. the partner no longer attends to hygiene as when they were dating, there is less communication, or the sexual experience feels like a mechanical act). These can often be dealt with through communication, although both parties may need to accept the idea that they could hear things that are less than flattering.

A low-sex relationship can often deteriorate so that conflict, frustration, and boredom become commonplace in the relationship. With education, communication, and proper motivation, however, these relationships can usually re-establish a healthy sexual life together.

Maintaining sexual desire, attraction, and trust is an ongoing process that takes effort and initiative for both individuals. When a couple's sexual expression begins to lag and lack excitement, the key to rebuilding marital sexual desire is to increase intimacy and joy together.

Successful relationships are all about a good fit. One person may want sex once a month while the other person wants it every evening. Which one has a problem? Most likely neither. The point is that someone who wants sex less than their partner does not necessarily have low sex drive that needs to be treated. If it feels low to the person (i.e. a change from what they are normally experiencing), then perhaps they might seek some help. If it is simply not at the level of their partner, it may be more likely to be a problem with sexual compatibility. In those cases, couples can learn to find common ground and compromise. In rare cases, the incompatibility may be insurmountable and the relationship cannot continue.

Many people are embarrassed to mention that their low sex drive may be due to no longer being attracted to their partner. They feel that sex should not be important to them and so feel guilty about these thoughts. This is in fact very common. Sex is important in a relationship, and being attracted to one's partner is also important. Should we tell our partner to lose weight and then we will be attracted to them? "Letting oneself go" may be perceived by the other person as disrespectful/being taken for granted, and it may be difficult to feel sexual when being disrespected. In addition, we often find someone attractive because they have a certain level of self-respect, and not attending to weight, health, or hygiene may come across as a lack of self-respect. Attraction is not simply about appearance. Some people lose attraction for their partner because the person has become unsupportive and so they are seen as less attractive. Can you get the attraction back? Depending on why it has been lost or diminished, couples should spend more time together, talk more (e.g. try to recall why you initially found the person attractive and try to communicate what has been lost), and even schedule sexual intimacy.

What if it is not even that clear? What if "something seems to be missing" in the relationship? Discussing these issues as a couple can be very difficult but seems essential if the relationship is to continue on a healthy path. Professional help may be useful in these situations so that discussions on these topics do not degenerate into blaming and saying hurtful things in moments of frustration.

Low sexual desire can have a multitude of causes, and this chapter can hardly do service to all of these possible causes. These might include childhood sexual abuse, guilt regarding previous sexual activities or partners, religious issues, body image preoccupations, fears of failure, fears of pregnancy or difficulties such as infertility, fears of abandonment, shame about a sexual fetish, the need to protect a partner, or a lack of genuine feelings for one's partner. For an individual with medical concerns or chronic health problems, additional issues may play a role in the lack of sexual desire. These might include shame or negative feelings about one's body, concerns of being a burden, fears of rejection, the work involved in preparing for sex, fatigue, lack of privacy, difficulty with erections or ejaculation, and feeling inadequate as a sexual partner. These "secrets" often affect the trust in a relationship and can seriously impair communication. Ideally, they should be discussed with one's partner or at the very least with a therapist, best friend, or sibling.

Nutrition, Diet, and Sexual Drive

Many people wonder if something they are eating or drinking may result in a low sexual drive or, conversely, increase sex drive. Many vitamins and supplements have been speculated to have effects on sexual desire – mainly by the people selling them. Nicotine and alcohol may lower sexual drive by reducing blood flow in the genitals (discussed above), but no natural supplements have been reliably shown to reduce sexual drive. Interestingly, no supplements have been shown to increase sexual drive either, despite years of lore and myths of aphrodisiacs.

In terms of dietary issues, again we have no reliable data that diets rich or deficient in certain vitamins/minerals have a positive or negative effect on sexual drive. Foods that promote heart health, however, can indirectly assist in sexual performance, possibly because they improve genital blood flow. As sexual performance improves it makes sense that we would want more sexual activity. Conversely, foods that negatively affect our heart may make physical exercise (and therefore sexual activity) difficult, and this in turn may make us less interested in pursuing sexual activities. Additionally, high-fat foods may make us feel and look overweight and unattractive, and therefore make us (or our partner) less interested in sex. One can see that these dietary issues are rather indirect links between diet and sexual drive, but there is no evidence for more direct effects between foods and sexual drive. Some foods/drinks such as those containing caffeine that produce energy may lead us to direct our energy toward sexual activity, but again there is no link that caffeine directly makes us more sexual.

Many people are concerned about the effects of marijuana on sexual desire. There is an amotivational (i.e. motivational deficit) syndrome that may accompany marijuana, often after a period of chronic (extended) use. The lack of motivation may appear the same as low sexual drive, but the key difference is that the lack of motivation from marijuana extends beyond sex and may show itself as loss of motivation to undertake a range of activities including socializing, personal hygiene, and so on.

Sleep and Low Sexual Desire

Poor sleep or lack of sleep can lead to low energy, fatigue, and sleepiness. These factors can in turn affect libido and lead to a decreased interest in sex. The combination of low energy and increased tension caused by lack of sleep can also lead to sexual dysfunction.

Men with obstructive sleep apnea (OSA), an inability to breathe properly during sleep, commonly report low libidos and sexual activity. OSA has also been associated with lower testosterone levels in some men. OSA is also associated with sexual dysfunction in women.

Finally, people who have trouble sleeping often develop elaborate bedtime routines. One of the things that can disturb sleep is a bed partner and so they may sleep separately from their partner. Sleeping in separate beds or bedrooms often leads to less sexual activity, which in turn may lead to less desire for sex and negatively affect the relationship. If this is the case, speaking with each other about the issue and arranging "protected intimate time" together can help.

Learning to improve sleep, either through lifestyle changes such as reducing caffeine (especially after midday), keeping the bedroom dark, quiet, and somewhat cool, or using cognitive therapy may improve sexual drive. Less commonly, having a sleep evaluation may inform the person about OSA or other sleep disorders affecting quality of life.

Genetics of Sexual Drive

Many people wonder if low sexual drive is genetic. A few years ago, scientists in Israel found a common genetic trait that seems to be associated with an increased sex drive, a gene known as dopamine D4 receptor (*DRD4*), which partly controls the brain's response to dopamine, a chemical associated with the body's reward system. Scientists know that this neurotransmitter plays a role in sexual behavior in animals and humans, and that dopamine circuits underlie the drive for things such as sex, drugs, and food. Because dopamine has many functions in the brain that influence behavior, it is unclear how this gene is associated with libido. The gene may be more appropriately related to a person's desire for seeking novel situations and behaviors. Discussion of genes in sexual drive is interesting, but it is more likely that an array of different genes subtly mold our sexual desire and behavior, along with cultural expectations, upbringing, and life experiences. There is not a single "pro-sex" or "anti-sex" gene.

Myths about Sexual Desire

Two common myths about sexual desire are that heterosexuals have lower sexual drives than homosexuals and that frequent masturbation results in low sexual desire. As to the first, there is no evidence that gay people have higher sexual drives. This myth may be due to the fact that sex for gay men may culturally be easier to access or due to the anti-gay propaganda that many espouse that gay men are hypersexual and therefore perverts. Although this myth has many interpretations and possible etiologies, there is no credible evidence that sexual orientation is associated with different intensities of sexual drive.

As to the second point, many worry that frequent masturbation makes them enjoy sex less when with another person and so they become less sexual. Masturbation may refocus sexual desire on certain behaviors that the person cannot find when with another person. Masturbation to pornography may also fuel the self-focused quality of a person and so when they have to accommodate another person when having sex, this may feel difficult, alien, or even uncomfortable. Therefore, frequent masturbation may indirectly lead to less sexual drive directed at another person. How much masturbation is too much, or who might be affected by this, however, is not known. Ideally, a person should learn to marry their masturbation life with their sexual life with other people. This may take practice. In some cases, professional counseling may assist the person to transition from the self-focused world of masturbation to the otherness of sex with a partner. That does not mean eliminating masturbation but simply reducing it perhaps to accommodate someone else.

Sexual Anorexia

Sexual anorexia has been described as an obsessive state in which the physical, mental, and emotional task of avoiding sex dominates a person's life. The individual is obsessed with avoiding sex and finds it repulsive. This differs from having a low libido or being simply not interested in sex. Thus, sexual anorexia is different from having low sexual desire. Those with low sexual drives do not avoid sex; they have difficulties activating their libido. They simply lack interest, as their desire has been squelched or is nonexistent. They may be avoiding a partner who wants sex more than they do, but they also seek to avoid confronting their own low desire. The concept of sexual anorexia dates back to the 1970s, but there are still no credible data regarding how common this condition is.

Sexual anorexia takes on many forms: a pattern of resistance to any sexual topic or overture; continuing that pattern of avoidance, even though the person knows it is destructive to the relationship and might drive their partner away; going to great lengths to avoid a partner's sexual contact or affectionate attentions; rigid or judgmental attitudes toward sexuality and the physical body; and obsessing over sex and how to avoid it, to a point where it interferes with normal living. The sexual anorexic's main goal is to find ways to separate intimacy and sex. Men and women alike can suffer from sexual anorexia, but it should be noted that it is not currently a recognized mental health condition but rather a description of what some people experience.

Treatment of Low Sexual Desire

Assuming the above-mentioned medical issues have been examined and there does not appear to be a cause of the low sexual desire such as those listed above, then psychological therapies, such as cognitive behavioral therapy (CBT), may help. If a relationship issue is at the heart of the problem, the best treatment for low sexual desire in either partner is counseling to resolve overt conflicts, hidden resentments, power struggles, or other interpersonal barriers to erotic interest.

Perhaps the most effective route is educating both men and women about how women and men actually become aroused. One treatment of low sexual desire in women uses mindfulness to connect bodily sensations of arousal with psychological arousal.

There is no magic pill for restoring sexual desire among women or men, nor is there likely to be. In men, a drop in testosterone levels can profoundly impact sexual desire, and, especially as men age, treatment with testosterone may restore desire. Male hormones, such as testosterone, play an important role in female sexual function, even though testosterone occurs in much lower amounts in women. Replacing testosterone in women is controversial and it is not approved by the US Food and Drug Administration (FDA) for sexual dysfunction in women. In addition, it can cause acne, excess body hair, and mood or personality changes. Estrogen delivered throughout your whole body (systemic) by a pill, patch, spray, or gel can have a positive effect on brain function and mood factors that affect sexual response. But systemic estrogen therapy may have risks for certain women. Smaller doses of estrogen – in the form of a vaginal cream or a slow-releasing suppository or ring that you place in your vagina – can increase blood flow to the vagina and help improve desire without the risks associated with systemic estrogen. In some cases, your doctor may prescribe a combination of estrogen and progesterone.

Originally developed as an antidepressant, flibanserin is a prescription medication approved by the FDA as a treatment for low sexual desire in premenopausal women. Sometimes referred to as the 'female Viagra,' flibanserin may boost sex drive in women who experience low sexual desire and who find the experience distressing. Flibanserin appears to increase dopamine and norepinephrine levels and decrease serotonin levels in the prefrontal cortex. Potentially serious side effects include low blood pressure, dizziness, and fainting, particularly if the drug is mixed with alcohol. Experts recommend that you stop taking the drug if you do not notice an improvement in your sex drive after 8 weeks.

When to Ask for Help

This chapter has shown that low sexual desire runs a spectrum from some symptoms to an actual disorder called HSDD. The take-away point is that if your level of sexual desire is troubling you in some way, you should discuss it with your primary/family doctor. It may be that simple education from your primary physician regarding sex or intimate relationships might be useful, or that some physical health issue is impacting your sexual desire and can be addressed quickly and easily. You will not know unless you ask about the issue. Too often, people wait until a problem is large before asking for help, and this can make the solution to the problem more difficult or more time consuming. Also, this is about your quality of life, and that should be important. Having said that, your doctor may not be able to fix the problem, but they may know other possible resources (e.g. psychological counseling) that could be beneficial.

Summary

This chapter has described many facets of low sexual behavior. To better summarize the main points, we return to the cases of Theresa and Stewart. These cases show that many variables can influence the presentation of low sexual drive (e.g. relationship stress) and that in turn low sexual drive results in many other issues for the person (e.g. body image, self-esteem). At some point, these become circular, and it is difficult to tell what is cause and what is effect. Many issues surrounding low sexual drive can be dealt with through lifestyle changes, health changes, or talking with one's partner(s). In cases where the low sexual drive is causing more significant problems, professional counseling is warranted.

6 Too Much Sex

Cheryl is a 42-year-old heterosexual female and has been married to her husband for the past 23 years with whom she has two high-school children. Over the past year, Cheryl has been showing increasingly prominent symptoms of depression, spending long periods of time secluded from the family and struggling to complete her work as an accountant. After urging from her husband, Cheryl agreed to see a psychologist about her depression and problems with work. While meeting with the therapist, Cheryl noted that she has been feeling increasingly depressed, attributing this to feelings that she is an immoral person. Upon further inquiry, Cheryl revealed that she has had affairs with different men throughout her married life, and that this behavior has increased in frequency over the past several years. In fact, she describes almost weekly sexual contacts. Some of the affairs have been one-night stands, while others have continued for a few weeks. Cheryl admits that the affairs are "purely sexual." She loves her husband and has no intention of leaving the marriage. She enjoys the "thrill" of finding partners on the Internet and enjoys the passion. She would like to consider herself a moral person, however, and so this behavior is particularly troubling to her, as it is contrary to what she believes her moral nature to be. As a result, Cheryl started feeling increasingly helpless and guilty about her behavior, describing her compulsive sexual behavior as "immoral" and her inability to control it a "personal weakness." The almost constant preoccupations with sex intrude upon her work life and have made her less productive and more prone to errors. Cheryl also notes that she hasn't told her husband about her problem because she worries that he will leave her and take the children. Cheryl emphasizes that although she enjoys the sexual behavior, she wants to stop it before it causes more problems with her work and family, but she doesn't know how to control her urges, thus leading to escalating feelings of depression and despair.

Reggie is a 28-year-old gay man who reports that he exclusively has sex with other men, as both a receptive and a penetrative partner. During an appointment with his primary care physician, Reggie reported that he had been experiencing notable pain while urinating and had noticed discharge from his penis during the previous week. Following several tests, the doctor confirmed that Reggie had contracted gonorrhea, likely from a recent sexual partner. While discussing the treatment for gonorrhea with Reggie, his doctor also made a point of asking him about the types of protection he uses during sex and how many partners he has had recently. After being asked the additional questions, Reggie started to explain that he had been struggling to control his urges to go cruising over the last couple of months and had started having sex with large numbers of partners he met at local bars and clubs, with whom he had almost entirely stopped using protection. Reggie described his cruising behavior as "out of control," and described how he felt there was almost nothing he could do to stop himself from engaging in risky sex with partners he met. He also emphasized that while he often felt it was fun to meet partners, he also felt increasingly worried about the possible consequences of his behavior, and felt highly distressed that the behavior felt like it was out of control.

Too Much Sexual Desire

The idea of extreme or out-of-control sexual desire has been written about for centuries, and yet this has continued to be a topic of some debate. Despite being discussed and treated by many mental health professionals, the American Psychiatric Association (APA) recently refused to officially recognize this behavior as a psychiatric disorder, as they felt that there was not convincing evidence for its existence and that even the idea of it was too vague. Although the APA did not acknowledge excessive sexual desire as an independent disorder, the World Health Organization (WHO) has recommended it be included in the 11th edition of the *International Classification of Diseases*. The WHO felt that diagnoses that impact public health should be recognized. Excessive sexual desire is associated with sexually transmitted infections including HIV infection, unintended pregnancies, viewing of pornography at home and in the workplace, and extensive cybersex users who use the Internet for seeking partners.

As shown in the cases above, we do know that many people struggle with sexual desires that feel out of control. So how do we explain or harmonize these two positions? The lack of convincing scientific evidence for excessive sexual desire does not mean it does not exist, it simply means that we currently cannot clearly define the biology of the behavior. The same could be said of depression. The difference is that depression has already been recognized and so does not meet the same skepticism as a "new" behavior. The bottom line is that a lack of convincing scientific evidence for the cause of excessive sexual desire does not mean it is not real or deserving of attention. In many areas of medicine, the problem is recognized first and the cause is found out later.

Excessive Sexual Drive Has Been a Recognized Problem for Centuries

Although it is difficult to compare possible historical notions of excessive sexual desire, some forms of the behavior appear to date back centuries. The first medical accounts that we have found date back to 1775. The idea of excessive sexual desire has gone by many names over the years, and people may be confused by the various terms for this behavior that they can find on the Internet. The terms "nymphomania" and "satyriasis" (for females and males, respectively) date back to the eighteenth century to describe people who engaged in premarital intercourse or reported erotic fantasies. More recently, terms such as sex addiction, hypersexuality, excessive sexuality, or problematic sexual behavior have all been used in the popular media to refer to this excessive sexual drive.

Compulsive Sexual Behavior

For this book, we have chosen the term "compulsive sexual behavior" (CSB) to refer to the condition of having too much sexual drive, as it aptly describes the behavior without suggesting any judgment regarding the behavior. The term CSB characterizes repetitive and intense preoccupations with sexual fantasies, urges, and behaviors that are either distressing to the individual (due to the out-of-control nature of these thoughts) and/or result in some type of impairment, such as poor work performance or interpersonal issues. Individuals with CSB often perceive their sexual behavior to be excessive and are unable to control it. They act out impulsively (act on impulses and lack impulse control) or compulsively (are plagued by intrusive obsessive thoughts and driven behaviors).

To make the diagnosis of CSB, an individual must endorse recurrent and intense sexual fantasies, sexual urges, and sexual behavior that results in some impairment in functioning and at least one of the following four symptoms during the same 6-month period:

1. The person is preoccupied with some aspect of sexuality or being overly sexually active.
2. The person has repetitive sexual fantasies that feel out of control or cause distress.
3. The person has repetitive sexual urges that feel out of control or cause distress.
4. The person engages in repetitive sexual behavior that feels out of control or causes distress.

It is important to recognize that there are multiple behaviors that are encompassed by the term CSB. There are at least seven common behaviors: compulsive cruising and multiple partners, compulsive fixation on an unattainable partner, compulsive autoeroticism (masturbation), compulsive use of erotica, compulsive use of the Internet for sexual purposes, compulsive multiple love relationships, and compulsive sexuality in a relationship.

Evaluating the prevalence of CSB is difficult, due to the embarrassment and shame frequently reported by those with CSB and society's judgmental position toward the expression of sexuality. Although no large epidemiological studies have been performed, the estimated prevalence rate of CSB is approximately 3–6 percent. One recent study of public university students found that 2.0 percent (3.0 percent for men and 1.2 percent for women) met the diagnostic criteria for CSB.

Most people who struggle with CSB are reluctant to mention it to their clinicians, and most clinicians are generally uncomfortable talking about sex with their patients due, in part, to a lack of training. It is more likely that a person will bring the topic up when they are being treated for a sexually transmitted infection, an unwanted pregnancy, or marital or relationship problems. Other people might present with anxiety, depression, or alcohol or drug use problems, and in these cases, the sexual behavior may be driving these issues (e.g. the person drinks to cope with their out-of-control sexual behavior), may be the result of these other problems (e.g. a person is depressed and the only way to "self-medicate" the depression is by seeking the excitement and high from sex), or is often simply co-occurring with these other conditions.

Excessive Interest in Sex

Overpathologizing sexual behavior can occur by failing to recognize the wide range of normal human sexual expression – in frequency but also in variety. This can also occur among family members and clinicians who possess overly conservative attitudes and values regarding sexual expression. It is important for people who feel they have CSB to find a professional they are comfortable discussing a wide range of sexual behavior with, and they should consider seeking consultation from a specialist in sexual health. Patients who see a clinician who is uneducated about sexuality may end up feeling more embarrassment and shame than prior to the appointment.

Sometimes, individuals, with their own restrictive values, will diagnose themselves with this disorder, thus creating their own distress. Therefore, it is very important to distinguish between an individual who has a values conflict with their sexual behavior and those who engage in sexual behaviors that are driven by impulsive, obsessive, and/or compulsive mechanisms. For example, one man who came to our clinic did so because he masturbated once every few weeks but felt that any masturbation was "sinful and perverted." In this case, "treatment" consisted of simply educating him about the range of sexual behaviors that are normal and healthy.

There is an inherent danger in diagnosing CSB simply because someone's behavior does not fit the values of the individual, group, or society. There has been a long tradition of pathologizing behavior that is not normative within a culture. For example, masturbation, oral sex, homosexual behavior, viewing pornography, and having an extra-relational affair could be viewed as compulsive behaviors because someone might disapprove of these behaviors. There is no scientific merit, however, to viewing these behaviors as disordered, compulsive, or "deviant." When someone is distressed about these behaviors, they are most likely in conflict with their own or someone else's value system, rather than this being due to CSB.

Behaviors that are in conflict with someone's value system may be problematic but not necessarily out of the person's control. Sexual problems are often caused by a number of nonpathological factors. People may make mistakes, or they may lack awareness of the law. They may, at times, act rashly. Their behavior may cause problems in a relationship. Some people use sex as a coping mechanism similar to the use of alcohol, drugs, or eating. This pattern of sexual behavior may become problematic. Problematic sexual behavior is often remedied, however, by time, experience, education, or brief counseling.

Not All Excessive Sexual Behavior Is CSB

Just because someone is hypersexual does not mean that they have CSB. As we mentioned earlier, only about 3–6 percent of people in the general population would meet the criteria for

CSB. Therefore, when someone is excessively sexual, it is important to think about other possible reasons for the behavior. Other problems may result in a person becoming hypersexual. The first thing to keep in mind is that not all excessive sexual behavior equals CSB. As we mentioned above, sexual behaviors that are in conflict with someone's value system may feel problematic and even excessive but are not objectively so. Similarly, just because someone has more sex than someone else does not equate with CSB. The value system of the patient, the family, and even the clinician may get confused with CSB.

In addition, there are several other issues that often become confused with CSB when a person is overly sexual. For example, CSB must be distinguished from the excessive sexual behavior that is often seen in new relationships. In those situations, the excessive sexual behavior is usually time limited and does not typically cause distress or result in impairment. Of course, extreme cases of sexual behavior (e.g. masturbating six times a day and being unable to get to work on time due to the masturbation) are the more straightforward cases to diagnose. The difficulties are in the "gray area." Take the example of a young man who is unemployed and spends hours each day looking at pornography, which he finds hard to control and distressing because it upsets others. Is this CSB or simply a result of having excessive free time? This is where the above-listed diagnostic criteria can be very useful. It is also a simple question of how much control the young man has over his behavior. For example, if a job comes up and he can stop his behavior and function at a high level, then it probably is not CSB.

Excessive sexual behavior can occur as part of mania, as in the case of bipolar illness. A manic episode is when a person is out of control, feeling too euphoric (or being extremely irritable), and doing multiple impulsive behaviors that are getting them into trouble, for at least a week. For a manic episode to be diagnosed, the symptoms must not be due to direct effects of drugs on the brain. Sexual behavior may be one of those impulsive behaviors that some people get when having a manic episode. If the problematic sexual behavior also occurs when the person's mood is stable, the individual may have CSB in addition to bipolar disorder. This distinction is important because the treatment for bipolar disorder is very different from that for CSB.

Excessive sexual behavior can occur when a person is high on drugs. In particular, stimulants (e.g. cocaine, amphetamines) as well as gamma-hydroxybutyrate (GHB) may result in excessive sexual behavior. It has never been demonstrated whether these drugs are aphrodisiacs or whether they simply create so much excess energy that the person expels that energy sexually. Either way, the person using them may engage in excessive sexual behavior. If the sexual behavior does not occur when abstinent from drugs, then the appropriate diagnosis would likely not be CSB.

Finally, it is important to determine whether the person started being hypersexual after beginning any medications. Some patients taking certain medications (e.g. medications for Parkinson's disease or restless legs, aripiprazole for depression/psychosis, stimulants for attention deficit hyper-activity disorder) may experience excessive sexual behavior. These medications, for some individuals, may increase dopamine in specific parts of the brain involved in reward and control (see Chapter 3). If the sexual behavior decreases or stops when the medication is reduced in dosage or ceased, then a diagnosis of CSB would not be indicated, because the behavior was "secondary" to (i.e. due to) medication.

Clinical Aspects of CSB

The majority of individuals with CSB who seek treatment are men with onset of CSB during late adolescence. However, our case of Cheryl shows that women also struggle with CSB. In fact, one study of adolescents found that young girls were more likely to have CSB than young boys. In contrast, studies generally report higher rates in men and more severe symptoms in men. Clinicians are less likely to screen women for CSB as they often incorrectly see this as a disorder only affecting men. This bias may be due to cultural views of women and sexuality. Finally, even adolescents may struggle with CSB. We have seen cases of adolescents who seem to have behaviors similar to adults with CSB. One case in particular was seemingly triggered by the adolescent inadvertently seeing illegal pornographic versions of children's films on the Internet.

Individuals with CSB may cite certain mood states as triggers for the sexual behavior, most commonly sadness or depression, happiness, or loneliness. Furthermore, a majority of individuals with CSB may experience a dissociative state (a sense of feeling outside one's body or detached from the world) while participating in CSBs. After engaging in the behavior, most feel shame and experience a negative mood change, ranging in length from minutes to days. Even though the individuals dislike behaving and thinking in such a manner, it distracts them from other concerns, reduces anxiety or tension, improves mood, and makes them feel important, powerful, and excited in the short term.

Research has shown that individuals with CSB have an average of three different CSBs. The most commonly reported are masturbation, compulsive use of pornography, and protracted promiscuity/compulsive cruising and multiple relationships. The Internet is another avenue for CSB, because the Internet is available 24 hours a day, 7 days a week, is affordable, and is perceived to be anonymous. About 72 million people visit pornography websites annually, and research has shown that between 10 and 20 percent who use the Internet for sexual purposes have online sexual problems. Studies have shown that sexual compulsivity is strongly related to the amount of time spent pursuing online sexual activities. Online sexual activities include pornographic audio, video, and text stories, real-time chatting with fantasy partners, searching for a sex partner, replying to sex advertisements, purchasing sex products, and contacting prostitutes.

Risk Factors for Developing CSB

Both men and women can develop this problem. Most studies have found that the majority of individuals with CSB who seek treatment are male. Most individuals with CSB have onset of this illness during late adolescence. Due to the sensitive nature of sexual behavior, however, there is some suggestion that the prevalence of CSB may be underreported in the general population and that females may be underrepresented in these clinical samples. A recent study found that 3.1 percent of women who responded to an online survey were characterized as hypersexual. Another found that 5 percent of women reported having some problems with internet sexual behavior. These studies highlight the importance of bearing in mind that CSB can occur in both genders.

Several factors may influence the gender disparity in CSB. First, the majority of individuals seeking treatment for CSB are males and, compared with men, women experience more CSB-related shame. Second, research has found that, compared with females, males have more sexual fantasies, masturbate more frequently, become aroused more easily, and have more causal attitudes toward sex. Males also more commonly engage in sexual relations for pleasure and self-esteem reasons, whereas females more commonly participate in sexual relations to further their relationships and to develop long-term commitments. Another factor that may contribute to the perceived higher proportion of CSB in males is the cultural double standard that men who are highly sexual are labeled as being "men," while females who behave in a similar fashion are viewed as promiscuous.

Given that males and females often pursue sexual relations for differing reasons, it is possible that CSB presents differently in females. For many females, being in a relationship may be more enticing than the sexual activity. Women may therefore be more likely to engage in multiple

love relationships rather than compulsive cruising or multiple superficial partners.

A national study of risky behaviors among youth
in grades 9–12 in private and public US schools (i.e. aged
14–18 years) indicated that 47.8 percent of students had
had sexual intercourse, 7.1 percent of students had had
sexual intercourse before the age of 13 years, 14.9 percent
of students had had sexual intercourse with four or more
individuals in their lifetime, and 35.0 percent of students
had had sexual intercourse with at least one person
during the 3 months prior to the survey. With the
increased rates of sexual activity in this age range, will
we see more CSB as well? Little research has explored
the area of adolescent CSB. One study found that 4.9 percent of adolescents in a psychiatric inpatient unit had
a co-occurring diagnosis of CSB. To date, this is the only
known empirical study assessing rates of CSB within an
adolescent population and was limited to psychiatric
patients.

Studies measuring sexual compulsivity have identified that between 20 and 28 percent of LGBTQ individuals
score highly on sexual compulsivity measures. In addition,
men who have sex with men appear to have significantly
higher sexual compulsivity scores than women who have sex
with women. Some researchers have suggested that sexual
compulsivity may be more frequent in the gay and bisexual
male community due to the availability of gay-oriented
sexual outlets, such as sex parties, bathhouses, and sex
websites.

Sexual compulsivity has been associated with sexually risky behaviors in both homosexuals and heterosexuals. One study comparing gay men with inner-city, low-income heterosexual men and women found that sexual compulsivity was significantly associated with unprotected intercourse, total number of sexual partners, and sexual sensation seeking in both gay men and heterosexual individuals. Compared with heterosexual males and females, however, gay men were more likely to report inconsistent condom use and multiple sex partners.

Another study of 180 inner-city men self-identified as gay or bisexual with HIV found that, compared with those with low sexual compulsivity, men with high levels of sexual compulsivity were more likely to have unprotected intercourse and less likely to disclose their HIV status.

When asked about the reasons for their sexual compulsivity, gay and bisexual men cite both intrinsic (i.e. poor mental health, low self-esteem, need for validation and affection, stress reduction, and biological predisposition) and extrinsic (i.e. relationship issues, availability of sex, childhood sexual abuse, and maladjusted parental relationships) reasons as a source for their CSB. Other studies of CSB within the LGBTQ community have linked higher levels of internalized homophobia with greater sexual compulsivity.

Possible Causes of CSB

In terms of the family, substance use problems are common in the relatives of individuals with CSB. In a survey of individuals with CSB, most participants had experienced at least one substance addiction in their family. In fact, only 13 percent of individuals with CSB come from a family without a substance use disorder. How should we interpret these data? One interpretation is that CSB may have a familial or even a genetic link to substance addictions. Another interpretation, which is not mutually exclusive to the first, is that a certain chaotic family environment due to addictions may give rise to CSB.

Research suggests that the majority of individuals with CSB come from families that have stressful dynamics. Restrictive environments regarding sexuality and dysfunctional attitudes about sex and intimacy may contribute to the later development of CSB. One theory concerning CSB and family interactions suggests that, as a child, the overly sexual person's emotional needs were not met either because of parental rigidity or from lack of follow through, resulting in the child believing that people are unreliable and that they can only depend on themselves. Sex therefore becomes a source of well-being to these individuals.

Several studies have also linked the development of CSB to childhood abuse. Significant rates of emotional, sexual, and physical abuse have been found in individuals with CSB. Rates of childhood abuse in people with CSB may be three to four times higher than in people without CSB. Although causality between adult CSB and childhood experiences has not been established, an assessment of CSB may also warrant further investigation into an individual's familial relationships and developmental background.

From the medical perspective, the onset of CSB has been linked to a variety of conditions, including head traumas, brain surgeries, mental health illnesses, both prescription and nonprescription medications, frontal lobe lesions, temporal lobe epilepsy, dementia, multiple sclerosis, and the treatment of Parkinson's disease with dopamine drugs. However, most cases of CSB do not have a "known biological cause."

Several studies have examined serum testosterone and sexual activity in CSB. In adult males, testosterone is secreted in pulsatile fashion with the pulse height and frequency varying slightly throughout the day and at different times of the year. Research, however, suggests that frequency of sexual activity and level of sexual interest do not correlate with serum testosterone concentrations. However, other hormones may be involved (e.g. studies suggest that luteinizing hormone, produced in the pituitary gland, may play a role in excessive sexual drive, but the data are very preliminary).

In terms of cognitive functioning, research findings have been inconsistent. One study found maladaptive cognitive processes and perceptions about sex in a population of homosexual and bisexual men compared with heterosexual men. A different study with heterosexual, homosexual, and bisexual men found additional potential cognitive differences where hypersexuality, being more impulsive, and experiencing negative emotions were all associated with lower mindfulness (less being present in the moment). Another study in people with CSB found that they did not differ from those without CSB in terms of cognition, although the sample size was fairly small.

Brain scans of people with CSB have produced interesting findings, but it is unclear how, if at all, we can use the information to help people with CSB. When presented with cues of varying sexual content, individuals with CSB reported greater sexual desire and the cues resulted in increased brain activity in areas associated with desire and emotions, the same regions implicated in studies examining triggers to drug cravings.

Consequences of CSB

Individuals with CSB may face a variety of medical complications including but not limited to: unwanted pregnancies, sexually transmitted infections, HIV/AIDS, and physical injuries due to repetitive sexual activities (e.g. anal and vaginal trauma, burns/damage from overuse of a vibrator).

A major health risk for those with CSB includes sexually transmitted infections, such as HIV/AIDS. Higher levels of sexual compulsivity appear to be related to more unprotected sexual acts, a higher total number of sexual partners, and being diagnosed with multiple sexually transmitted infections. A study of HIV-positive individuals found that, compared with those who were not sexually compulsive, people with CSB were significantly more likely to report engaging in unprotected vaginal or anal intercourse, having more total sexual partners, and engaging in sexual behaviors that could lead to HIV transmission. In addition, four times as many new HIV infections can be expected in the HIV-negative partners of sexually compulsive individuals.

Individuals with CSB report that significant marital, occupational, and financial difficulties are consequences of their sexual urges and behaviors, and that significant distress is caused by the amount of time spent consumed by their urges, thoughts, behaviors, out-of-control feelings, and post-behavior guilt. Mental health consequences, such as anxiety and depression, are common in CSB.

Although studies have documented the connection between substance use and sexual behaviors, few have specifically examined the connection between CSB and substance use. Substances can alter the experience of sexual behaviors. Methamphetamine increases drive, and many report that it heightens sexual desire and sensations, while decreasing sexual inhibition, while cocaine leads to feelings of well-being, self-confidence, and alertness. Research has shown that substance abuse is common in individuals with CSB, but the temporal relationship is not always clear. Did the person become addicted to drugs because they were initially looking for sex and drugs came along with the sexual activity, or did the sexual activity get out of control due to the drug addiction?

The substance abuse–sex connection may be stronger among gay men, because substance users typically feel more confident and desirable, and have an easier time cruising for sex and making contact with another person, resulting in greater success in finding a partner. One study examining drug use in African-American men who have sex with other men found that drug use facilitated feelings of hypersexuality or sexual compulsion, increased comfort with approaching other men, and allowed them to cope with feelings of homophobia.

CSB and Deviancy

CSB is not the same as a paraphilia (a term used to describe more unusual sexual behavior that has been judgmentally referred to as perversion). CSB involves normative sexual behavior, while the paraphilias involve sexual behavior that is socially anomalous or that is historically considered deviant. A paraphilia is a condition in which men or women are compulsively responsive to, and dependent upon, an unusual and personally or socially unacceptable stimulus.

Paraphilias may involve illegal behavior such as an adult having sex with a minor. Not all sexual offenses, however, are committed by people meeting diagnostic criteria for a paraphilia. Examples of paraphilic disorders are: pedophilia (interest in children), exhibitionism (exposing oneself), voyeurism (watching others in sexual situations), sexual sadism (humiliating others), sexual masochism (being humiliated), fetishism (finding an object sexual), and frotteurism (rubbing against people for sexual pleasure).

Treatment of CSB

The first step in treatment of CSB begins with an accurate diagnosis. To make an accurate diagnosis, it is important first to rule out medical causes of CSB. Certain neurological disorders can cause an individual to act inappropriately and possibly result in CSB. Some of the most common examples are Alzheimer's disease (causes sexual disinhibition due to the effects of the disease on the frontal and temporal lobes, with a prevalence of between 4.3 and 9.0 percent of patients), Pick's disease (impairs the regulation of socially acceptable behaviors) and Kleine–Levin syndrome (causing hypersomnia, which can cause abnormal behavior such as hypersexuality). In addition, certain types of medications or illicit drugs can result in an increased sexual drive such as dopamine agonists used to treat Parkinson's disease, or cocaine, GHB, and methamphetamine.

When CSB is suspected, the patient and family members are advised to find a specialist in this area for assessment and treatment. For example, in the USA, resources include the American Association of Sex Educators, Counselors and Therapists (www.aasect.org) and the Society for Sex Therapy and Research (https://sstarnet.org).

Sometimes, people simply need to understand the patterns of their behavior and the negative consequences, and be more motivated to engage in sexually healthier behaviors. In cases where individuals feel that normative sexual behavior is somehow pathological, the clinician can educate the individual about the normative range of sexual expression. Disagreements in value systems between couples are also common. These disagreements can be acknowledged, and the couple can work to find compromise solutions for handling their disparate value systems, as is done with value conflicts in raising children, family relationships, or managing finances.

It is also important to recognize that some people with CSB simply get better on their own. Known as "natural recovery," this occurs in many addictions, as well as in CSB. It is unclear, however, who can ultimately control their behavior without any interventions. Some data suggest that mild cases of the disorder and those early on in the course of illness have better potential for natural recovery. One thought is that these individuals are actually performing a type of therapy on themselves. The idea of correcting cognitive distortions and substituting healthy behaviors in place of previous problematic sexual behavior is not unknown to people even without therapy. Although natural recovery may occur, on the individual level, the possibility for it needs to be balanced by the current levels of distress and dysfunction of the person.

There are also some special issues in treatment. Several common situations may influence the treatment approach to someone with CSB. If there is active substance use such as crystal methamphetamine, the question is whether the person can be treated as an outpatient and whether the same approach can be used for the substance addiction as well as for CSB. There are instances where the substance use interferes with CSB treatment, and the individual may need to be referred for detoxification or residential placement for the drug addiction before receiving therapy focusing on CSB.

When an individual with CSB also exhibits clear signs of mania, this needs to be addressed. The mania will need to be treated before the person can take full advantage of the treatment for CSB; indeed, the CSB may resolve (or become less severe) with treatment of the manic episode. In most cases, treatment for the mania will involve medication to stabilize the person's mood.

In cases where individuals with CSB have significant personality disorders such as narcissistic personality disorder, the standard treatment plan for CSB may need to be modified to include more psychodynamic approaches.

Psychotherapy for Excessive Sexual Behavior

In many cases, psychotherapy is helpful for CSB. CSB is often deeply rooted and can stem from a lack of usual psychosexual development. Many people with CSB have grown up in challenging family environments and have underlying identity and intimacy problems. Many may have lacked nurturance, love, acceptance, and positive role models. As a result, their psychosexual development has been adversely affected, and this has ultimately prevented them from feeling good about themselves as sexual beings and resulted in problems with intimacy.

One of us was trained in the treatment of CSB by Dr. Eli Colman's group at the University of Minnesota's Program on Human Sexuality. Although controlled studies in psychotherapy for CSB are lacking, expert clinicians have been treating individuals with CSB for many years. Based on these years of experience, the preferred modality in that facility was group therapy combined with additional individual and family therapy. Weekly group therapy is useful to examine how a person learns from the coping strategies of others and develops new intimacy skills. Group therapy reduces the intense feelings of shame due to the sexual behavior. Using an ongoing group, new members are able to learn from others who have almost completed and are able to understand the whole course of therapy. The group also provides peer support for improved coping.

Individual therapy, often involving a mix of CBT, supportive therapy, and dynamic analysis, allows the therapist to address personal issues in greater depth. Individual therapy also allows issues to be addressed as they arise in groups. Family therapy focuses on family of origin issues and conflicts in interpersonal functioning. Family therapy can also focus on rebuilding trust within relationships, as this is often damaged by a person's sexual behavior.

Goals of Treating Excessive Sexual Behavior

A goal of therapy is to work toward gaining some control over the problematic sexual behavior. To start, it is practical to focus on controlling the most problematic sexual behaviors such as those that increase the risk for serious health problems such as HIV. The individual with CSB should understand that this process takes time. Given the generally impulsive nature of many people with CSB, the idea of taking time to gradually gain control over one's behavior may be unsatisfying and may be the reason for dropping out of treatment. Therefore, the patient and therapist should set realistic goals at the beginning of therapy. One other issue is that, due to the shame of the behavior, many patients will set unrealistically rigid goals for themselves, such as "no masturbation ever." Some of this is driven by overly restrictive sexual attitudes about sexual expression, which may have been one of the driving forces initially behind the CSB, and may also be motivated by a need to feel good about oneself. The problem is that it can backfire when the goal is too rigid and unrealistic. In addition, the person needs to learn how to accept themselves and their sexual feelings and to feel good about themselves, independent of their sexual behavior.

Because the goal of treating excessive sexual behavior realistically cannot very often be abstinence, the person needs to be able to define sexual boundaries of acceptable and unacceptable behavior. This is an important process between the clinician and patient. The patient must be involved in setting these boundaries, and a consensus should be established between the clinician and patient. The role of the therapist is to challenge overly restrictive or overly liberal boundaries. The next step is to set goals for staying within those agreed-upon boundaries, such as describing sexual behaviors that are within and outside the boundaries.

Many people are quite distressed when trying not to engage in their sexual behaviors. Some feel like they cannot cope with distress or that they grieve the loss of their best friend (much like someone with alcoholism may refer to the bottle as their best friend). This may lead to feeling anxious or depressed. Coping with these feelings in therapy is important, as they could lead to relapse if not dealt with effectively.

As CSB often reflects an underlying disturbance in identity and intimacy, another goal of therapy is to develop a healthier understanding of oneself as an intimate being.

This understanding of oneself may require addressing body image issues, which often arise in treatment. Many individuals with CSB are deeply insecure about their appearance and whether they are attractive. Those with CSB are often used to developing a fleetingly good sense of oneself: "If they have sex with me, then I must be attractive." Cognitive therapy focusing on perceived attractiveness is often used to deal with these concerns.

To address problems with intimacy, as well as to identify cognitive distortions that maintain CSB, patients are often asked to write their sexual autobiographies that include information about their history of sexual activities such as age of first sexual behavior, history of intimate relationships, and problematic or traumatic sexual experiences. Patterns of behavior are discussed and maladaptive patterns addressed. Recognizing these patterns allows the person to develop an understanding of situations or emotional states that may trigger their CSB. They can then recognize a sequence of events that lead to their CSB and perpetuate it. By understanding the cycle, the person can learn to interrupt it. Relapse prevention strategies are used for this purpose.

Medication for Excessive Sexual Behavior

Medication can often be helpful in reducing CSB urges and behaviors. Many people, however, may be resistant to the idea of medication. Education focusing on the possible biological causes of CSB, as well as the side effects and possible benefits of medication, may make the use of medication more appealing. Patients should be informed that there have been very few randomized clinical trials and that mostly we depend upon expert opinion. None of the medications that we use now is FDA approved for CSB, which means that any medications we use are referred to as "off-label" (i.e. they have been approved for some other health problem but not for CSB). In addition, medication may in fact make psychotherapy more beneficial. Therapy often transiently provokes anxiety or depression, and medications may help with the emotional response to therapy.

The most frequently used medications for CSB are the selective serotonin reuptake inhibitors (SSRIs), a class of antidepressant medications. These medications have been shown to be quite effective in treating depression and anxiety, and, at the same time, are often helpful for CSB. These medications also seem to help with some aspects of impulse control, and their primary side effect is decreased libido, which can help in controlling CSBs. When used for CSB, SSRIs may be useful in reducing the desire for sex, frequency of masturbation, and hours of pornography use per week. One potential caveat of SSRIs is that, with some people, a decreased ability to have an orgasm may result in more extreme problematic sexual behaviors. For these people, the riskiness of the sexual behavior may be ramped up to override the sexual side effects. This would be a case where the medication needs to be used in combination with therapy.

Naltrexone, an opioid antagonist approved for treating alcoholism and opiate addiction, has also shown benefit in treating CSB. Naltrexone has been effective in reducing urges in similar behavioral addictions and in reducing relapse in alcohol and opiate addiction. Not only does naltrexone seem to reduce the sensation and pleasure-seeking aspects of the behavior, it may also be helpful for aspects of impulsivity.

Lithium and anti-epileptics may also provide some benefit in CSB. These medications have been used in the past and still remain potentially effective treatments. In some patients in which SSRIs are insufficient in controlling their CSB, these medications can be used instead of or in addition to an SSRI; however, these medications often have more side effects.

Finally, in more resistant cases, anti-androgens can be used. These medications control libido and help with sexual urges. There are much more severe side effects to be considered, but they remain a potentially useful medication option when other interventions do not work.

Support Groups for CSB

Sex Addicts Anonymous (SAA) is an example of a support group whose purpose is to help those with sex addiction find recovery. This organization operates similarly to Alcoholics Anonymous (AA) with a focus on the 12-step program. Another support group available to individuals is Sex and Love Addicts Anonymous (SLAA), which is also similar to both SAA and AA. There are no data regarding how well people do when attending SAA or SLAA, and so we advise individuals to use individual or group therapy and then use these support groups as augmentation.

Summary

This chapter has described many facets of excessive sexual behavior. To summarize the main points, we would like to present another representative case. Michael is a 24-year-old gay man who has been sexually active for almost 10 years. He has multiple partners each day as it helps him feel good about himself: "I feel attractive and wanted when someone has sex with me." His behavior has placed him in several dangerous situations where he has been robbed and raped. He is also currently concerned that he may have contracted HIV from a recent sexual act.

Michael started group therapy for CSB. Initially uncomfortable being gay in a group with many heterosexual men, he gradually grew to enjoy the support. In addition, he was started on naltrexone to reduce his sexual urges so that he could take part in the group discussions more effectively. "The medication helped me to be able to focus on what other people were saying in the group whereas before I found myself constantly thinking about sex." In individual therapy, Michael focused on body image issues and intimacy problems.

Over the course of the next 12 months, Michael continued to do well. He was able to set boundaries of acceptable and unacceptable sexual behaviors and stick within those boundaries. He had a negative HIV test. The fear of getting HIV has continued to be a motivating factor in his care.

7   Sex and Physical Health

Audrey is a nursing student who has always focused on work rather than having a boyfriend. She seldom masturbates as she feels guilty when she does and thinks it could be abnormal. At her 21st birthday party, she finds two friends making out in a bedroom. Audrey begins to ponder her own situation of being single and the young men she has dated occasionally but never taken it to the "next level" with. She has heard that unprotected sex can lead to sexually transmitted infections, or unplanned pregnancy, but she wonders if she is missing out – she wonders if there are any positive benefits of sex, rather than it being "all bad" or just for the purposes of having children.

James is a 50-year-old man with long-term diabetes, who had a heart attack 2 years ago while he was out running in a local marathon. Following the heart attack, he made a good recovery but is understandably nervous about putting too much strain on his heart, in case something similar happens again. He has started running again because his cardiologist said this would be safe for his heart, but the cardiologist didn't say sex was safe. James has avoided sexual intercourse with his wife, Charlotte, since leaving the hospital. Charlotte has accepted this because she does not want James to worry, but she has felt more emotionally distant from James because sex was previously very important in their relationship.

The possible negative effects of sexual activities are frequently discussed – sexually transmitted diseases and unplanned pregnancies are important public health consequences of sex when excessive or not conducted with appropriate planning (e.g. with use of barrier contraception). Societies also propagate myths about the negative effects of sex, which are not backed up by any sound evidence, such as the idea that too much sexual intercourse can cause strokes, or that masturbation will make you blind and result in hair growing on your palms. Historically, issues of sex and sexuality were taboo, and this remains the case, albeit to a lesser extent than before. The risks of sex have been quite well studied, but the potential benefits of sex are far less studied in research – and when research finds benefits of sex, these results are less talked about because they are perceived as taboo or embarrassing. Because sex involves orchestrated, complex activities, it can be affected by physical health conditions. Like Audrey in our case example above, many people have been taught about the dangers of sex but have not necessarily thought about, or been taught about, what positive consequences it might have.

In this chapter, we first consider whether there is evidence that sex can be good for us, before then considering physical health issues and sex – with a special focus on heart problems and diabetes as examples.

Sex and Physical Health

Generally, anything that exercises our heart can theoretically be seen as a good thing, because it strengthens the heart muscle and has other positive health benefits including reducing cholesterol levels, blood pressure, and the risk of diabetes. Because sex is a form of exercise, it also burns calories and fat. So, if a person has regular sex, do they need other exercise? Research shows that the heart rate during sex, for most people, is similar to levels that would happen during light exercise such as a brisk walk. In young adults, sex can be as energetic as moderate exercise rather than light exercise. Nonetheless, you are unlikely to be meeting your recommended total exercise time per week with sex, especially as the average length of time for sexual intercourse in one large survey was 5.5 minutes. There is another reason not to use sex as your only form of exercise: a study following 80 men over a year found that doing regular nonsex-related aerobic exercise was linked with improvements in sexual performance and sexual satisfaction.

In Wales, in the UK, information was collected over 10 years from 1,000 men aged 45–59 years. The men were asked how often they had sexual intercourse, and had regular medical check-ups that included measurement of blood pressure, monitoring of cholesterol levels, and a trace of the heart's electrical activity. At the end of 10 years, men who had at least two episodes of sexual intercourse per week had half the risk of having died compared with men who had sexual intercourse less than once per month. Of course, there could be differences between these two groups that could explain this, rather than the risk of death being reduced by sex. The authors also ran a statistical analysis to control for age, smoking, and social class, and still found a significant association between more sex and lower risk of premature death. Some have criticized the findings, arguing that the link between sex and reduced risk of death could be explained by other variables that were not recorded. This is theoretically possible, but this criticism can be levied against any study of this type. If we accept that more frequent sex might protect against early death, what might explain this?

The study in Wales also reported that more sexual intercourse (twice or more per week) was additionally associated with a lower risk of fatal heart attacks compared with people who had less sexual intercourse. Sex frequency, however, did not affect the risk of having a stroke. So, sex might be good for the heart, which in turn might reduce the risk of early death.

In a Swedish study in 300 older people, men who stopped having sexual intercourse earlier in life had a higher risk of death, but no significant protective effect of sex was found for women.

In the USA, a study in North Carolina followed 250 people over 25 years. The women in the study who had more enjoyment of intercourse in the longer term had longer life expectancy, while for men, a higher frequency of intercourse predicted longevity. Again, this hints at protective effects of sex and/or sexual enjoyment on health but does not prove the causative link.

How could we convince the naysayers and prove that sex can have positive effects on heart health and life expectancy? The only way to do this would be to conduct a controlled clinical trial in which we randomized people to have regular sex or no sex over several years (we doubt many people would agree to enroll!). This simply is not realistic or ethical, so we will have to make our own conclusions based on the evidence. The studies above show that more frequent sex is associated with better heart health and less risk of early death in some groups of people, but they only hint at sex itself being protective, rather than proving it.

Could sexual activities be protective against some types of cancer? As discussed in Chapter 4, a couple of studies have shown an association between a higher frequency of masturbation (or ejaculations) in men and a lower risk of prostate cancer. In France, a study was run in about 50 women who had been diagnosed with breast cancer and in a control group of 95 women who did not have breast cancer but were otherwise similar (e.g. in terms of age). Risk of breast cancer was associated with having sexual intercourse infrequently and with having no sex partner. There is also evidence that having children and breastfeeding may be associated with a lower risk of breast cancer. One possible explanation for this is that hormonal factors can influence cancer risk. For example, regular sex could lead to increased oxytocin (the "love" hormone mentioned in Chapter 3) and DHEA (dehydroepiandrosterone, a steroid-related hormone that is normally present in humans), which might in turn protect against breast cancer, because these hormones regulate how cells in the body develop and grow.

Anecdotally, patients often tell us that sex helps with sleep and relaxation. Many people report a good night's sleep after sexual activity. When having an orgasm, there is a surge of endorphins and oxytocin, chemicals that can lead to bonding and relief of tension. In several anonymous surveys, more than 20–40 percent of people reported using sex or masturbation to relax and to help with sleep. Fifty men and women were asked to fill in diaries about sexual activities over a 2-week period, and were exposed to stress in the form of public speaking and doing mental arithmetic. Recent sexual intercourse was associated with a better stress response – their blood pressure went up less during the stress. Interestingly, recent masturbation (whether self-masturbation or mutual masturbation) did not seem to have this beneficial effect. Sex seems better than masturbation for stress relief!

A reduction in our stress response, however, is not just about sex. In other research, 70 women in a long-term relationship were told that they would need to give a 5-minute mock job interview followed by completion of difficult arithmetic in front of strangers. This is a form of the famous Trier Social Stress Test, a reliable way of stressing out unfortunate study participants under standard laboratory conditions. Before doing these stressful activities, the participants were randomized to have 10 minutes' worth of physical contact with their partner (massage), verbal-only contact with their partner, or no contact with their partner. They then did the mock interview and arithmetic. Those who received physical contact from their partner before the stress test had better stress responses: their cortisol levels (cortisol is a key chemical released in response to stress) and heart rates did not increase as much as expected. Those who received verbal-only support from their partner did not differ from those who received no contact, in terms of their stress responses. When asked about how stressed they felt following the experience, the groups did not differ from each other. In other words, close physical contact with our partner before stressful events can help reduce the consequences of stress on the body, without us even being aware of it. We may feel just as subjectively stressed as we would otherwise, but our blood pressure and stress hormones do not seem to respond as much.

Sex may reduce pain perception. Laboratory studies have demonstrated that sexual stimulation and orgasm make us able to tolerate higher levels of pain (i.e. they increase our pain threshold), at least temporarily – although most research has been in women rather than in men. This has led to speculation that sexual activities could help with pain, such as in arthritis, menstrual cramps, migraine, or spinal injuries. There is some evidence for this, but the topic is understudied. In a survey of migraine sufferers, most people who had experienced migraine symptoms reported that sex improved migraine (even ending it completely) if they had sex during a migraine. However, these benefits did not seem to extend to people with cluster headaches. Migraine typically involves feeling sick (or even vomiting), finding exposure to light or noise uncomfortable, and visual disturbances such as seeing strange halos or lights, whereas a cluster headache typically involves a one-sided headache, watery eyes, and a runny nose. Why sex seems to help migraines but not cluster headaches is anyone's guess, but it might be that different biological processes underlie these two types of headache.

Finally, could sex make you more youthful? The jury is out. One study found that more frequent sexual intercourse was linked with looking younger (even 7–12 years younger!) compared with people with less frequent sexual intercourse. This was found in both men and women. Of course, we cannot say that the one caused the other.

Sex and Mental Health

If sex is good for the body (e.g. the cardiovascular system), as seems to be the case, could it also be good for the brain? The brain is a greedy organ – it requires a lot of nutrition and oxygen. Because the cardiovascular system supplies these to the brain, improving it could in turn help brain function. Additionally, because sexual intercourse lowers our physiological responses to stress (e.g. cortisol release, blood pressure), this in turn could be beneficial for the brain. Evidence in humans and nonhumans shows that chronic stress has multiple negative effects including suppression of the immune system, increased risk of infections (e.g. lung infections), and a tendency to retain more fat in our bodies, leading to obesity. These negative effects of stress are at least partly due to the impact of stress on cortisol and other chemical signaling pathways. Chronic stress over time also leads to changes in several brain regions, including the hippocampus (involved in memory) and the frontal cortex (involved in regulating our desires; see Chapter 3). These effects of stress on key brain regions might be why stress can lead to escalation of comfort-seeking behaviors such as comfort eating, shopping, or excessive masturbation.

There is recent evidence that sex might help some aspects of brain function, especially as we get older. In a UK study of approximately 7,000 adults aged 50–89 years, participants were asked about their sexual activities over the past year and did a memory test. They heard a list of 10 everyday words and were asked to recall them straight away and then again after a short delay. More frequent sexual activity in the past year was associated with better memory performance on the task, in both women and men. This is interesting given the negative impact of stress on the hippocampus in the brain, which is involved in memory, and would certainly be important in allowing people to recall items. In men, there were some additional apparent benefits of sexual activities: better performance on a number sequencing task, which is linked with the function of the prefrontal cortex. Sexual activity included masturbation, petting, and intercourse, all included under one category, so it was not possible to say whether some types of sexual activities seemed more strongly related to these apparent beneficial brain effects than others.

Satisfaction with our sex lives is highly correlated with quality of life. In a US study of 3,500 men and women, personal happiness was related to the frequency of sexual activities and orgasms, while another US survey of 500 men and women found widespread beliefs that a satisfying sex life is important for quality of life across the age span. Earlier sexual satisfaction seems related to sexual satisfaction in later life – so satisfaction in adulthood makes it more likely we will also be satisfied as we get older. Of course, sexual satisfaction is not always the same as quantity of sex; the goal for satisfaction is that the amount of sex is right for us, or for our relationship situation.

In fact, given personal preferences regarding frequency of sex, it is not surprising that a higher quality of life has been associated with personal satisfaction regarding one's sexual life. Monks who eschew sexual relations for religious reasons can have a high quality of life and low stress levels. Someone who craves sex, is socially isolated, and cannot get a date might have a low quality of life and high stress levels. People with some types of personality might be content being celibate. In a National Epidemiologic Survey in the USA, in around 35,000 adult men and women, around 1 percent reported never having had sexual intercourse. Did these people have high rates of mental health problems? In fact, celibate individuals compared with others were less likely to have substance use disorder and some other mental health problems. However, the members of the celibate group were more likely to have certain personality types (avoidant and dependent personality) and obesity. It looks like "horses for courses" (and "courses for horses"). Depending on the type of people we are and a host of other factors, we may be comfortable with a certain level of sexual contact with others. Provided our actual sexual experiences are not too different from what we are comfortable with on an individual level, sex or a lack of it is not likely to have a negative effect on our quality of life and might improve it.

Sex during Pregnancy

Pregnant women and their partners worry about whether sex is safe in pregnancy or could have a negative effect on the baby such as increasing the risk of miscarriage or harming the unborn baby. In fact, penile–vaginal sex and masturbation are safe for most pregnant women and their unborn child. If a pregnant woman is at risk of miscarriage (or has had miscarriages in the past), at risk for preterm labor, experiences vaginal bleeding/discharge/cramping, has a condition called placenta previa (a rare condition in which the placenta covers the opening of the cervix), or is expecting multiple babies (e.g. twins, triplets), then they should speak with a healthcare professional for advice before having sex during pregnancy. This advice applies not just to sexual intercourse but also potentially to other types of sexual activity. Also, if the male or female has a sexually transmitted infection, then having sex during pregnancy can in some cases lead to the infection being passed on to the baby (when the baby is in the womb and/or during delivery). For these reasons, it is sensible to check for sexually transmitted infections through a family doctor if you have any concerns (both partners), ideally in advance of trying to become pregnant, and to discuss any such risks with your healthcare professional in advance.

Under normal conditions, the baby is physically protected in the uterus by amniotic fluid and by the woman's cervix, so penile thrusting into the vagina will not cause discomfort or distress to the unborn child, unless (potentially) there are medical issues as listed above. Pregnancy brings with it a host of changes to the woman's body, and sexual desire will often (but not always) reduce during some time periods of the pregnancy. Pregnancy can bring with it not just hormonal changes but also emotional changes, tiredness, nausea, breast tenderness, weight gain, and back pain – any of which could affect sex.

Most sexual positions are fine during pregnancy, although a couple may find some sexual positions (e.g. lying together on their sides) more comfortable. If considering anal sex during pregnancy, this can be fine, but be aware that pregnancy can increase the risk of having hemorrhoids and of constipation – anal sex can be more painful and may lead to bleeding if there are hemorrhoids.

In addition to fluctuations in sexual desire during pregnancy, it is not uncommon for a female partner also to notice changes in their male partner's attitude toward sex. Some men worry about "poking the baby" and so are reluctant to engage in sexual activity, or they experience performance anxiety. As long as there is none of the conditions listed above, sex during pregnancy is generally safe and so there is no need to worry. Theoretically, sexual intercourse leading to orgasm could trigger labor earlier than expected if a woman is very close to giving birth (late in the third trimester). However, when a survey asked women about sexual activities they undertook close to delivery dates, there was no evidence that premature delivery was significantly higher when intercourse was undertaken close to delivery.

Sex and Heart Problems

In the case vignette, we described James, who had a heart attack 2 years ago and has avoided sex with his wife ever since because he was worried about the risks. Sexual activity is a common worry for people who have had a heart attack or other types of heart disease. While doctors should always talk with patients about this matter following a new heart-related diagnosis, most of the time they do not, and patients are reluctant to bring up the topic. During sexual activity, the biggest changes in our heart rates and blood pressure happen around the time of orgasm, and these usually return to normal a few minutes after the conclusion of sex. When healthy volunteers agreed to have their pulse and blood pressure recorded during different sexual activities, it was found that man-on-top sex and woman-on-top sex were associated with similar increases in pulse and blood pressure, but the men expended more calories with the first type of scenario. Several research teams have compared pulse and blood pressure changes during sex with those observed during other forms of exercise. In general, they found that the changes in pulse and blood pressure during sex were no greater than during some types of exercise, such as climbing two flights of stairs or going on a brisk walk.

Bearing this in mind, should James, who had a heart attack during a marathon 2 years ago, be worried that sex with his wife will cause another heart attack? It is understandable that he would be worried about this, but, if he can do other daily activities without experiencing chest pain or shortness of breath, such as climbing two flights of stairs or taking a brisk walk, then he is probably fine to take part in normal sexual activities. The same advice applies for a woman who has had a heart attack. Under these circumstances, the risk of having a heart attack during sex with a partner is most likely no different from someone who has never had a heart attack. James should continue with any treatment and advice discussed with his doctor following the heart attack, such as watching what he eats, and not doing more strenuous activities (such as running) without professional healthcare advice first. Importantly, using alcohol or illicit drugs in conjunction with sex, eating a heavy meal within 3 hours of sex, or having sex at a stressful time would increase the risk, and so sex should be avoided at these times. Also, extramarital sex could be more hazardous for someone who had a previous heart attack than having sex with one's usual partner – extramarital sex is more likely to involve use of alcohol/drugs, having sex after a heavy meal, or more extreme types of sexual practices, all of which could increase the risk.

What about other heart problems? Some people experience chest pain and have a diagnosis of coronary artery disease (narrowing of the arteries supplying the heart muscle) but have never had a heart attack. Other people have unusual rhythms of the heart, or problems with the valves in the heart. Again, we advocate a sensible approach: provided the individual does not have cardiovascular symptoms (e.g. chest pain, shortness of breath) during regular activities of taking a brisk walk or climbing two flights of stairs, regular sex is likely to be fine. It is good to follow the principle of "start low and go slow," rather than starting with intense and lengthy sexual activity. Once a person is comfortable with lighter sexual activities and knows they did not have any cardiovascular symptoms, they can build up to full normal sexual activities. In case of any concerns, and certainly if any cardiac symptoms occur during sex or other activities, speak with a doctor for advice before doing it again. The bottom line is that decisions about sex should involve awareness of the benefits of sex but also of the risks.

Heart problems (cardiovascular disease) can be associated with sexual problems in both genders, including decreased libido, loss of interest in sex, or delayed/absent orgasms. Men with heart problems can have additional problems such as erectile dysfunction, priapism (when the erect penis does not return to its flaccid state), retrograde ejaculation (semen flowing back into the bladder rather than all out of the penis), and premature ejaculation. Women with heart problems can notice decreased vaginal lubrication and changes to their periods. Drugs can often be the culprit – some of the medications used to control blood pressure and the body's fluid levels (anti-hypertensive medications and diuretics) are quite commonly associated with sexual dysfunction, as are some of the drugs used to treat depression (e.g. SSRIs). The first step in addressing sexual dysfunction that happens with heart problems (and in general) is to speak with a doctor such as a family practitioner. This is important because there are many potential causes of sexual dysfunction, not just the heart condition itself. If a person sees a doctor and it looks likely that medication caused the sexual dysfunction, options to discuss with the professional can include switching to a different medication or (if appropriate) trying a lower dose of the established medication. Alternatively, it may be another medical condition that could be responsible for the sexual dysfunction, such as use of substances (e.g. alcohol) or psychological issues (e.g. stress, relationship difficulties).

Frequently, several factors can be responsible for sexual dysfunction, not just one thing. Different treatment options are available depending on the likely causes of the sexual dysfunction. For example, erectile dysfunction can be treated with medication, vacuum devices, injections, or, less often, surgery. Vaginal dryness can be treated with suitable lubrication, while priapism requires prompt medical attention by going to the emergency room. Premature ejaculation can be treated with a variety of sexual techniques and via medication (some of the class of serotonin reuptake inhibitors).

Sex and Diabetes

Diabetes is a medical condition in which the body struggles to maintain control over levels of glucose in the bloodstream. This can happen either because the pancreas, an organ responsible for making insulin, does not make enough insulin or because the person's body is insensitive to the effects of insulin, or a combination of the two. Sexual activities are safe in people with diabetes as long as they are feeling fine at the time of sex. However, unfortunately, diabetes is commonly associated with a loss of sex drive. A person may still think about sex (or masturbation), but this does not translate into physical desire or a desire to actually do the act. This disconnect between the mind and body can be especially frustrating. It can also be hard to explain to partners. In these situations, it can be helpful for the person to tell their partner that they still find them sexually attractive but are unable to act on that attraction. If diabetes is the cause of loss of libido, then often improving control of the diabetes with the help of a specialized diabetes team will lead to an improvement in sexual desire. If a person with diabetes notices a loss of libido, it is worth seeing a doctor and specifically mentioning this loss.

In some people, diabetes can lead to sexual problems even if there is no loss of desire, or there may be additional problems as well as a loss of desire. In men, diabetes can cause erectile dysfunction (difficulties getting and maintaining an erection) and retrograde ejaculation. In women, diabetes can lead to loss of vaginal lubrication and painful sexual intercourse. These difficulties are partly due to the damage to nerves in the body that is frequently seen in diabetes, called "diabetic neuropathy." In general (not just in people with diabetes), research has shown that cutting down on smoking and alcohol, losing weight if obese, and exercising more can be beneficial for reducing the risk of sexual dysfunction and loss of sexual desire.

Of men with diabetes, up to 75 percent may report difficulties with erectile dysfunction at some point. In fact, erectile dysfunction in men can be an early sign of diabetes, even if diabetes has not been diagnosed. There are, of course, multiple physical and psychological causes of erectile dysfunction. Milder erectile dysfunction can involve difficulties sustaining a full erection during intercourse, but intercourse is still partly possible. In severe erectile dysfunction, a person may be unable to get an erection at all. Both can be very embarrassing and frustrating. The man's partner might interpret a lack of sex as meaning they are no longer attractive to the man. Men who experience erectile dysfunction should speak with a healthcare professional to help rule out other causes and to be sure that the diabetes is well controlled through diet, exercise, and medication options. Typically, adult men experience spontaneous erections, such as during the night or upon waking from sleep. If this pattern has changed and spontaneous erections no longer happen, this can suggest that diabetes or another physical health cause is behind the sexual dysfunction. If a man still experiences spontaneous erections at the same previous rate but has sexual dysfunction when with a partner, this suggests that there might be psychological issues contributing, such as loss of confidence, stress, or conflict. Erectile dysfunction is treated with a variety of methods, including use of medication (phosphodiesterase inhibitor, e.g. Viagra), a vacuum pump ("penis pump"), injections, or sometimes an operation. Psychological counseling can help to address any psychological factors that could be contributing, as well as helping the person come to terms with the problem.

In men who develop retrograde ejaculation due to diabetes, they may notice that little or no semen is released when they masturbate, or that their urine is sometimes cloudy when they urinate after sexual activity. Retrograde ejaculation can develop because of diabetes but also due to certain medications, or if the man has had a previous operation to treat a urological condition. Retrograde ejaculation can cause low male fertility, so it might be detected if a couple are trying unsuccessfully to conceive. Retrograde ejaculation does not generally affect sexual desire or fulfillment, except if a man becomes worried or sensitive about the topic, or feels guilty if his partner does not get pregnant due to it. Not all retrograde ejaculation needs treatment. If it occurs due to diabetes, then improving diabetes control can help stop nerve damage progressing, but this is unlikely to fix the problem. Alternatively, if retrograde ejaculation is due to a medication and is bothersome, a doctor may switch the medication to an alternative or reduce the dose. There are some medication options that can be tried if the retrograde ejaculation is bothersome and is due to mild bladder or nerve problems. There are also separate types of treatment to help overcome infertility if the infertility is due to retrograde ejaculation (bear in mind that only around 1 percent of cases of infertility are due to this).

Loss of vaginal lubrication or painful vaginal sexual intercourse can happen in women with diabetes and can be due to the diabetes. But it can also happen in women with diabetes for reasons other than diabetes. For example, some cases of vaginal dryness are due to neuropathy (nerve damage) from diabetes, while others can be due to medications or psychological factors (e.g. stress or depression). Because diabetes increases the risk of infections, some women develop vaginal yeast infections, which can lead to dryness. Infections – not just vaginal infections but also urinary tract infections – can lead to painful intercourse. Loss of vaginal lubrication or painful intercourse can also happen if there are relationship difficulties or a mismatch in sex drive between two people that leads to conflict. Again, see a healthcare professional, such as a family doctor, and tell them what you have noticed, so that potential causes can be examined. Vaginal dryness can be treated with lubrication, while infections can be treated with topical antibiotic or oral antibiotic depending on the type. Contrary to popular belief, there is very little consistent evidence that cranberry juice helps to prevent or treat urinary tract infections.

Summary

While unprotected sex has a number of risks, including unplanned pregnancy and sexually transmitted infections, we have seen in this chapter that sexual activities seem to have a number of beneficial effects in terms of physical health and mental well-being. These apply to some people but not to all. Examples of possible benefits of sex include it being a type of mild exercise, helping with sleep, helping with migraines, helping with relaxation and stress relief, contributing to the strength of the "bond" in a couple, possibly reducing the risk of some types of cancer, and improving brain health in older age. Scientists need to study these areas more, as research has traditionally focused on the negative aspects of sex rather than the positive aspects.

Many medical conditions, substances, and medications can negatively affect sex drive and the physical ability to have sex. We have focused on examples of issues faced by people with heart problems and diabetes. There are many interventions for sex problems associated with physical health conditions and the two key starting points are being open with your partner about these difficulties and discussing them; and making an appointment to see a healthcare professional to talk openly about the problem.

If you know your partner is worried about a physical health condition that affects sexual desire or behaviors, it is good to offer to go to medical appointments with them, if they approve (whether to sit in the consultation or just travel together and sit outside). This might sound obvious, but many people do not offer! By offering to go to the appointment, the unaffected partner makes it more likely that their partner will seek help, but this also shows support and commitment. Try to be open with your healthcare provider about any sex problems that are bothering you – be this loss of sex desire, infections, discomfort during sex, vaginal dryness, or erectile dysfunction. In our experience, healthcare providers often do not ask about sexual health, for fear of embarrassing the patient or themselves, but it is better to mention it so that problems can be ruled out, rather than suffering in silence. In many cases, sexual problems are very treatable.

8   Drinking, Drugs, and Sex

Robert is a 32-year-old single man who has avoided serious dating for most of his adult life. He finds the process of going to bars uncomfortable and so drinks alcohol when he goes out. He also finds it easier to talk with women when he is slightly inebriated. The problem has been that he does not have control over his drinking and some alcohol moves quickly to too much alcohol. This has led to awkward moments waking up the next morning with women he does not know and he cannot recall what he did. He has made a fool of himself at bars, flirting with married women, and has worried that this may jeopardize his business career if anyone in his line of work were to see him act this way. He also reports not remembering the sexual experience and so he would like to drink enough to talk with women but not be intoxicated to the point of making poor choices or not enjoying sex.

Michael is a 21-year-old gay male who enjoys using crystal methamphetamine just before having sex. He reports that the drug makes him sustain his sexual performance better, gives him more energy, and makes him more popular sexually. He denies any drug problem, claiming that he does not use crystal meth when he is not having sex and so feels he can control his use. Recently, however, he noticed that he does not really enjoy sex without the use of drugs. He finds it difficult to have an erection and an orgasm when sober. Initially he found sex exciting and used crystal meth to enhance his sex life, but in fact, over time he reports that he has become a bit unsure what he likes more, the drugs or the sex.

Interest in sexual desire and its relationship to drugs and alcohol date back centuries. People have used drugs and alcohol in an attempt to enhance sexual desire, sexual desire has been negatively affected by drugs and alcohol, and drugs and alcohol often play some role, to varying degrees, in people's stories of their sexual desire. This chapter explores the complex relationships between sex, drugs, and alcohol, and tries to explain what drives these behaviors. It also considers the "what" and "when" in terms of people needing assistance with disentangling these behaviors.

Drugs and Alcohol, and Their Effects on Sexual Desire

This topic is important as there are many myths, as well as a fair amount of science, regarding the relationship of sex and drugs. A lot of people use a lot of different drugs, and a lot of people have sex. There is always someone who will tell you that drug X or Z enhanced their sexual performance or the quality of their sex. How much of that is true? And even if it is true, how much should or would someone want to risk to have a potentially better sexual experience?

People have mixed sex and drugs for centuries. A large study of approximately 22,000 adults in several countries found that 59 percent of men and 60 percent of women had sex after drinking, while 37 percent of men and 26 percent of women had sex after smoking marijuana. Yet, with all of this history, there remain many unanswered questions regarding the influence of drugs on sexual desire, and this is partly due to the fact that drugs affect people differently. In fact, the same drug may affect two people in diametrically opposite ways. We know this: we all know about "bad drunks", people who become unpleasant or even aggressive when intoxicated, whereas others might become quiet and introverted, or even sleep, when drunk. Drugs also may play a role in sexual assaults and make people unaware of what is happening to them sexually or unable to oppose someone else's sexual advances.

Research has shown that heroin, amphetamine, cocaine and MDMA (methylenedioxymethamphetamine or "ecstasy") all result in erectile dysfunction in about 30–40 percent of people who abuse these drugs. In addition, sexual desire is decreased in people who abuse these drugs. Some people, however, report that if they use them infrequently, these drugs may actually enhance sexual desire and performance, but it is often difficult for people to control their use of drugs without them becoming habit forming and thereby impairing their lives. Despite the science, the myths about these drugs may be more positive than the reality and thus make people want to try them to enhance their sex lives.

Stimulants

Probably the most talked-about drugs used for sex are stimulants such as amphetamines and cocaine, as these are often thought to be aphrodisiacs. These drugs are used by people from all social classes and ethnicities, and of all sexual orientations, specifically because people feel they will enhance sexual drive. People may describe the sex as more energized and their stamina more pronounced. The stimulants do have some biological aspects that make some of these stories accurate. Stimulants temporarily enhance the release of dopamine, the pleasure chemical, and norepinephrine, a chemical that enhances stamina, thus potentially making the person feel good, energized, and focused. But they also alter the way we make decisions and can lead to an overemphasis on personal desires and short-term outcomes, and may result in people making poor long-term decisions leading to risky, unsafe sex. These drugs increase our heart rates and blood pleasure, which can enhance physical sensation, but can lead to cardiac events. They can also result in agitation and nervousness that makes a person horribly uncomfortable. Some have suggested that the increased sexual activity in some people is simply a response to this uncomfortable feeling and a way to distract the person from it.

Not all stimulants are the same in their associations with sexual drive. They also differ based on which form of the drug is consumed and how they are taken. Cocaine does not stay in the system for long. In fact, cocaine's effects may last only an hour or so, whereas those of methamphetamine may last as long as 11 or 12 hours. In fact, methamphetamine users are more likely than cocaine users to report strong associations between their drug use and sexual behaviors.

The effects on sex can also be quite variable while taking stimulants. Some people may desire more sex and so they have extended periods of intercourse but have problems with orgasm. Also, over time, the drugs are commonly associated with erectile dysfunction and a decrease in sexual desire. Equally troublesome as the potential erectile dysfunction and decreased sex drive is that amphetamines seem to have negative long-term effects on the brain's pleasure receptors, thereby detracting from the ability to have a sober sex life. As in the case of Michael, this results in difficulty in a person's capacity to experience joy without drugs, a common problem among chronic crystal meth users. Another important consideration is that when people "come down" from stimulants they often experience unpleasant symptoms such as low mood or agitation, which are likely to lead to loss of interest in sex and reduced sexual performance, so the use of stimulants for many can be a double-edged sword.

Cannabis

Other drugs are also historically associated with sex drive. One of the more commonly used drugs for sexual purposes is cannabis. Some people describe cannabis as an aphrodisiac, enhancing sexual excitement, or as a relaxant, making them relaxed about sex. Interestingly, cannabis has also been associated with a loss of interest in sex and loss of motivation for sex. These inconsistent results may also suggest that sexual drive is affected differently based on the amount of cannabis consumed. The cannabinoid system of the brain, particularly in an area called the amygdala, seems to play a role in reactivity to stimuli, which in turn suggests a role in intensity of emotions such as those associated with sex. Based on this same understanding of the brain, cannabis may also increase fear and sadness and thereby make a person less sexual. Who will have one type of response or the other cannot be predicted. Additionally, research suggests that chronic cannabis use may result in decreased fertility and increased rates of erectile dysfunction. Unlike stimulants, however, cannabis does not appear to increase the riskiness of sexual activity. Dose may play a role in the mixed effects of cannabis on sexual desire: some studies suggest lower doses might facilitate sex, while higher doses impede it.

Ecstasy

Does ecstasy (MDMA) enhance sex drive? Ecstasy is a unique drug that seems to be a cross between an amphetamine and a hallucinogen. Reports suggest that ecstasy may increase sex drive, euphoria, and feelings of empathy. There is debate about whether the increased sex drive makes sense biologically given how the drug works. In addition, pure ecstasy might work differently in the brain from other types of ecstasy (it is frequently adulterated). This debate is further intensified by data showing that ecstasy may simultaneously increase sexual desire but also result in sexual dysfunction (e.g. erectile dysfunction).

Alcohol

Finally, and perhaps most importantly, we come to the role of alcohol in sexual desire. Alcohol is arguably the most commonly used drug for initiating or enhancing sex. Some research suggests that alcohol plays a role in over half of all sexual interactions in the USA, particularly in young adults. The story of Robert is a classic example of the complex interplay between alcohol and sex. Some anecdotes suggest that casual drinkers get a boost in sexual interest, arousal, or orgasm, while others detail problems with all of these. Research also suggests that drinking alcohol is associated with feeling more attractive and also finding others more attractive, known as "beer goggles."

Cognitive interference has been found to be a factor in sexual dysfunction in people who misuse alcohol. Alcohol affects a person's sexual arousal, control of arousal and rate of distractibility during sexual stimulation. They will fumble, have trouble focusing and may anger a partner during a sexual experience. This may lead to further problems with sexuality, as a person may begin to medicate their concerns with more alcohol. Indeed, alcohol impairs many aspects of cognitive abilities in a dose-dependent way, and this is why most societies have legal limits on blood alcohol consumption and being allowed to drive vehicles.

Alcohol can also reduce inhibition and negatively affect decision making, both of which can result in having sexual experiences that the person may not really want when sober. It can also lead to sexual experiences that are riskier and unprotected.

Males who drink alcohol may suffer from erectile dysfunction, a commonly reported side effect that has been found to be affected by age, mental health, and physical health. Conditions such as depression, anxiety, diabetes, and hypertension can all affect a man's ability to maintain an erection. Alcohol may factor into these related conditions as well. Alcohol is also known to prevent blood vessels in the penis from closing, inhibiting the ability of the penis to remain erect. In a healthy, nonalcoholic man, the penis becomes erect when aroused because it fills with blood and the vessels close, preventing back-flow. Chronic consumption of alcohol damages blood vessels, which causes problems in the heart and penis.

The psychological effects of alcohol on sexual performance should also be considered. Men often have high levels of guilt associated with poor relationships with partners, an inability to perform in the bedroom, and from not meeting expectations. Some men will medicate these feelings with more alcohol, which simply compounds the problems and leads to further feelings of inadequacy.

Women's sexual desires and experiences are known to be significantly impacted by alcohol. Many women state that they use alcohol to reduce their inhibitions, anxieties, and fears about sex. If this continues regularly, a woman may become dependent on alcohol to initiate or be involved in a sexual experience. Initially, alcohol can help a woman to be at ease with their body or the body of someone else, and to relax and enjoy a sexual experience. They will have improved confidence and well-being, which can mean positive sexual experiences. As drinking continues, however, its effects on the body, mind, and sexual desires will become apparent. Sexual desire will diminish, the ability to become aroused during sexual contact will be reduced, and many women will find it difficult to reach orgasm. In addition, alcohol can result in dehydration, and this in turn can result in lubrication problems for females, which may make intercourse more painful.

Women who use alcohol chronically may experience major physiological and psychological problems that affect sexual function. Problems with menstruation are common and, due to damage to the liver, the woman may be having hormonal changes that affect desire, arousal, and other sexual functions. Some women also experience physical changes such as vaginal atrophy or ovarian atrophy (changes in the growth of these types of tissue).

Stopping Drugs or Alcohol, and Sexual Desire

As is obvious from the above, drugs and alcohol often have negative effects on sexual desire as well as on sexual performance. That said, does it stand to reason that stopping the drug or alcohol use should improve or regain sexual desire? If that is true, how long should that take? The answers to these questions are not simple. Although we know that there are numerous health benefits when people quit (or reduce) using drugs or drinking alcohol, the sexual health benefits are less understood.

For years, people thought that men spontaneously recovered their normal sexual performance around 3 weeks after quitting substance use. Recent research, however, throws some of these older findings into doubt as it has found that drug use (alcohol, cocaine, heroin, or marijuana) negatively affects sexual performance in men even after a year of abstinence.

Treating the Sexual Issues Associated with Drugs or Alcohol

Should a person consider medication for erectile dysfunction secondary to drug or alcohol use? This becomes a complicated question quite quickly. Is the person experiencing sexual issues even after stopping the use of drugs or alcohol? Does it matter if the person stopped using drugs or alcohol? Should someone who uses drugs or alcohol still want to improve their sexual life?

There have been numerous warnings lately about the dangers of abuse of sildenafil (Viagra; as just one example of a medication for erectile dysfunction), and this seems to occur in cases where the medication is mixed with drugs such as ecstasy to enhance a feeling of euphoria and sexual excitement. One potential problem with this combination of prescription medication and drug is that mixing the two can trigger what is known as "serotonin syndrome," a condition where the person has too much serotonin, and this may result in confusion, disorientation, hallucinations, tremors, and, in severe cases, seizures, an irregular heartbeat, or even a coma. Medications for erectile dysfunction, such as sildenafil, are also often combined with "poppers", or amyl nitrate, for sexual enhancement. Both drugs dilate blood vessels and increase blood flow. This can result in a sudden drop in blood pressure, which can cause a stroke or heart attack.

Assuming, however, that the person is not using the erectile dysfunction pills to enhance sex by combining it with drugs of abuse, it may be warranted to consider it in the case of someone who has quit drugs or alcohol and is trying to regain their sexual performance. Because poor sexual performance may last for over a year and may result in poor self-esteem and even the choice to relapse to drugs or alcohol again, preventing these outcomes with medication for a short period of time may be worth considering.

Smoking and Sexual Desire

In addition to myriad health consequences, smoking may also negatively affect sexual desire. Several studies have found a link between smoking and difficulties having an erection. Nicotine is a vasoconstrictor, meaning it tightens blood vessels and restricts blood flow. In the long term, it has even been shown to cause permanent damage to arteries. As a man's erection depends on blood flow, the fact that studies have confirmed smoking's effects on erectile dysfunction is not surprising. In fact, one study found that just two cigarettes per day could cause softer erections in male smokers. Research has also demonstrated that men smoking more than 20 cigarettes a day (i.e. more than one pack) have a 60 percent higher risk of erectile dysfunction compared with their peers who do not smoke. Obviously, smoking is considered just one cause of erectile dysfunction. Others include stress, hypertension, alcoholism, diabetes, and prostate surgery. Young smokers may not notice the negative effects right away, but this could change over time and with chronic smoking.

Research has found that smoking significantly diminishes a man's sexual desire and satisfaction – even for young men in their 20s and 30s. Smokers who have partners report having sex less than six times a month, whereas nonsmoking men have sex nearly twice as often. Smoking appears to decrease sexual performance. When the ability to have sex decreases, the desire for sex will generally follow. Additionally, diminished desire appears to be combined with impaired performance in smokers, and this leads to decreased overall sexual satisfaction. When asked to rate their satisfaction with the sex they were having on a scale of 1–10, nonsmoking couples averaged 8.7, while couples with male smokers had an average of only 5.2.

There is far less research on the effects of smoking on women's sexual health. Some findings to date suggest that there may not be an increased risk of sexual difficulties among female smokers; however, nicotine dependence in women might be associated with lower libido. During sexual arousal, the labia, clitoris, and vagina also swell up with blood, similar to a man's penis, enhancing sensation and excitement. If nicotine can restrict blood flow and cause erectile dysfunction in men, it may be reasonable to predict that blood flow is restricted in women as well, and may also have a negative effect on sensation.

It is not clear whether sexual desire will improve once a person quits smoking, as there are many factors influencing sexual desire other than genital blood flow. Quitting smoking improves dental health (reduces stained teeth, better breath) and skin health (skin looks healthier, fewer facial wrinkles), and this might indirectly improve sexual desire through better self-esteem and a greater desire to be sexual.

Effects of Prescription Drugs on Sexual Desire

Several types of prescription drugs can result in sexual side effects, the most common of which are low sexual drive and difficulties with sexual performance (e.g. lack of orgasm, loss of erection). The list is large, so we have included some of the more commonly used medications. However, this list is not exhaustive and it does not mean that taking one of these medications will definitely result in sexual side effects. Sexual side effects have been reported with the following medications:

- Many, but not all, antidepressants, including older antidepressants (e.g. amitriptyline [Elavil], doxepin [Sinequan], imipramine [Tofranil], and nortriptyline [Aventyl, Pamelor]), as well as newer ones such as SSRIs (fluoxetine [Prozac], sertraline [Zoloft], and paroxetine [Paxil]) and selective noradrenergic reuptake inhibitors (venlafaxine [Effexor] and duloxetine [Cymbalta]).
- Antipsychotic medications: thioridazine (Mellaril), thiothixene (Navane), and haloperidol (Haldol).

- Drugs used to treat bipolar disorder: lithium and valproic acid.
- Anti-hypertensive medications (used to treat high blood pressure): spironolactone (Aldactone), thiazides (Diuril, Naturetin), methyldopa (Aldomet), reserpine (Serpasil, Raudixin), α-adrenergic blockers (prazosin [Minipress] and terazosin [Hytrin]), and β-adrenergic blockers (propranolol [Inderal] and metoprolol [Lopressor]).

There are also some prescription drugs that have been reported as resulting in hypersexuality. Some people may initially think this is useful, but the reports of the hypersexual behavior are not of people simply enjoying sex more; rather, they are of people who felt that their sexual behavior was largely out of control and that they were engaging in dangerous or inappropriate sexual behavior or engaging it in when they did not really want to do so. These side effects have interestingly resulted in lawsuits, and so the data regarding them are somewhat confusing and possibly colored by the legal issues (e.g. people may exaggerate symptoms if they want to sue a company). It is also interesting that people have tended to sue when their sexual behavior is out of control but not when the drugs described above have reduced or eliminated their sexual drive.

The drugs that have received the most attention have been those used to treat Parkinson's disease or restless legs. These drugs are known as dopamine agonists and, as discussed in Chapter 6, increasing dopamine has been linked with increased sexual drive. What was interesting about

161

these cases was that approximately only 10 percent of people taking them had behavioral problems. This raises two important issues:

1. Why didn't everyone taking these medications become hypersexual?
2. Some people gambled or drank more alcohol while only a few became hypersexual, so why didn't a person do all of these behaviors?

It seems that dopamine alone may not be enough. In fact, genetic predisposition and personal biology as well as personal developmental issues may play large roles in the development of hypersexuality or other behavioral issues. Furthermore, we do not yet know why one person may be hypersexual while someone else drinks too much. What is unique about the specific behaviors we gravitate toward is still unknown.

The other drug that has been implicated in making some people hypersexual is aripiprazole. This is an antipsychotic medication also widely used to treat depression. In a very small number of people worldwide, it seems to be associated with becoming hypersexual. This may have something to do with the fact that it too increases dopamine in the reward center of the brain. If it were that simple, however, why wouldn't more people or everyone taking it become hypersexual? We do not know, but it definitely suggests that if the drug plays some role, it is likely to be a fairly small one in the development of hypersexuality.

Natural Supplements and Sexual Drive

Humans have seemingly been in pursuit of an aphrodisiac for centuries. This has led to many tall tales about how various natural remedies result in longer love making, greater orgasms, and increased sexual desire. For all of these claims, however, there have been no credible studies proving that anything is truly an aphrodisiac.

All sorts of natural options have been bandied about online and on television as sexual enhancers. Some common ones include zinc (pumpkin), l-arginine, rhodiola *(Rhodiola rosea)*, folate (asparagus), and ginseng. The natural supplements that are recommended have some related conceivably credible theories, as most can theoretically increase blood flow, affect dopamine, or modulate sex hormones. Therefore, they seem to make sense as options. The real problem is that there is simply so little rigorous research supporting their use as sexual enhancers capable of increasing sexual drive. They might work for a few people, but without scientific research, we do not know who might benefit, to what extent the person may benefit, and why. One related exception might be maca root *(Lepidium meyenii)*, which has shown some mixed results in controlled trials of humans who experienced sexual dysfunction secondary to antidepressants. Another one shown to improve female sexual desire and arousal (in women with sexual dysfunction) in a meta-analysis was *Tribulus terrestris*. Similarly, a study found that fenugreek (*Trigonella foenum-graecum*) improved sexual desire and arousal in women with low sexual drive, while yet another meta-analysis found that saffron improved sexual dysfunction in both men and women.

Improving sexual drive when there is low drive or improving sexual dysfunction may not be equivalent to being a sexual enhancer, however.

Remember that the FDA does not require supplements to prove that they are safe, effective, or contain what they say on the label. You may want to look for a seal of approval from groups that check on supplement ingredients if you are considering using a supplement (whether for sex or anything else). These include the US Pharmacopeial Convention (USP) and NSF International. Note that vitamins and supplements are expensive and people can waste a great deal of money chasing after the elusive aphrodisiac.

Additionally, just because something is "all natural" does not mean it is safe. There are plenty of poisons in nature. A supplement may not be safe for a particular person depending upon their health issues and other medications they are taking. Some supplements can interact with prescribed medications, so it is important to discuss this with your doctor in advance of starting a new supplement, or medication if you are already taking a supplement. Finally, just because one pill of a supplement may be useful does not mean that taking a handful will be better or still safe. Always let your doctor know what you take in case it could affect your health or any medications that you take.

Drugs, Alcohol, and Intimacy

Sexual desire for many people is part of a larger relationship of intimacy. Intimacy often refers to close interpersonal relationships that usually involve both physical and emotional elements. The emotional component of intimacy is often the closeness that people feel for one another, whereas the physical component refers to sexual or romantic desires. Alcohol and drugs may have no negative effects on intimacy, but misuse or addiction to alcohol or drugs can. If people are abusing alcohol and drugs, then it can be almost impossible for them to maintain intimate relationships. This is because these substances often become their obsession, and there may be no room for anyone else. As the individual falls further into addiction, they may even lose their interest in sex completely. Addiction often results in the partner being unable to trust the addicted individual, and this too becomes a barrier to intimacy.

Drugs, Alcohol, and Body Image

How we feel about ourselves and our bodies may play a role in our level of sexual desire. The effects of drugs and alcohol on body image may therefore also work indirectly to affect sexual desire. The link between drugs and sex may not be direct but instead may be mediated through issues surrounding body image. The links between body image and drug use may be bidirectional. Some drugs can produce issues with body image (alcohol or smoking causing unhealthy-looking skin), while body image concerns may promote drug use (e.g. smoking or using stimulants to stay thin) as a means of coping with poor self-image.

For example, people often like stimulants for their weight loss properties. These drugs decrease appetite and increase metabolism, thereby potentially resulting in weight loss. The feeling of improved body image can augment the desire for sex, as people feel more attractive and desirable. In such cases, people are obviously making some decision about the balance between a perceived improvement to their body image versus the potential health issues of these drugs and even the negative sexual aspects to these drugs.

A similar conflict may underlie the use of nicotine. Many people feel that smoking cigarettes keeps them from eating and keeps them slim. A person may choose to smoke, despite the negative sexual aspects of smoking outlined above (sexual dysfunction, decreased desire). In addition, recent research suggests that men who start smoking when they are younger may actually reduce the size of their penises over time as a result of damage to blood vessels and penile tissue. Smaller penis size, especially if a man was used to a larger size before, can have numerous psychological effects on a man's self-esteem.

The case of opiates poses an interesting problem in terms of body image concerns. In extreme cases of body image, a person may actually have a condition referred to as body dysmorphic disorder, which is a preoccupation or obsession with some aspect of their appearance, and the preoccupation results in significant distress or functional impairment. People with body dysmorphic disorder tend to struggle with drug and alcohol addiction at rates far greater than the population at large. In our experience, people with this severely disabling condition report some improvement in the intensity of their body image obsessions with the use of opiates. We believe some people gravitate toward the use and misuse of opiates because of severe body image problems, and they find relief in the use of opiates. These men and woman should be educated about the fact that both therapy (CBT) and medications (anti-depressants) may be better and healthier options to deal with these body image issues.

Summary

This chapter has described the complex interrelationships between drugs, alcohol, and sexual desire. In the case of drugs, there are actually arguments that some of these chemicals may help improve sexual desire for some individuals. They come at a price to health, however. Perhaps the significance of these findings is that it may tell us how to utilize knowledge about these drugs to ultimately create a compound that could enhance sexual drive without the potential downside of addiction. In terms of alcohol and smoking, however, there is less evidence that these drugs have benefit for people in terms of sexual desire. Of course, drugs and alcohol have intricate connections to other aspects of sexuality such as health, body image, and emotional intimacy. Thus, it is difficult to know on an individual level how these factors interrelate. People are more complicated than just sexual desire, and so there are no easy answers about the relationship between drugs and alcohol and desire. Therefore, in the case of Michael we might suggest stopping crystal meth to allow him to reinvigorate his sexual life without drugs, whereas in Robert's case, perhaps he could reduce his drinking and learn to be comfortable sexually without having to jeopardize his health, or he could eliminate alcohol completely from his life but in a gradual way. The individual cases are difficult, and suggestions should be tailored based on the person, with professional healthcare advice.

9 Relationship Problems

Elton is a 37-year-old single man who recently got married after dating Erica for 3 years. During the dating period, he felt that sex was good but that they did not have it as often as he would like. Now having been married for 6 months, Elton has realized that nothing has changed. He would like to have intercourse at least four to five times per week, but Erica has expressed interest in sex only a couple of times during the entire 6-month period. Elton has made gestures toward sex but does not know how to talk about it directly. He worries that he may look like a "sex pervert" if he expresses his concerns. The lack of sexual relations, how-ever, has resulted in irritation on his part and feelings of insecurity. He finds himself easier to anger at his wife, having fights over silly little things, being less kind to her in general, and then feeling horrible about his behavior.

Stephen is a 41-year-old gay man who has just started dating Nick, someone he met at work. After the first two dates, the relationship became sexual. Stephen generally likes oral sex and avoids anal intercourse as it is simply not an activity he enjoys. Nick has told him that he really does not like sex unless there is anal intercourse. He and Stephen are attracted to each other, have lots in common, and find each other funny and interesting. After a month of dating, neither one is sure if they should continue the relationship. Nick feels unfulfilled sexually. He is growing

> *to care about Stephen and has discussed sex with him but feels that Stephen is unwilling to expand his sexual activities. Stephen feels the request is unreasonable, that there is more about a relationship than sex, and that Nick is prioritizing sexual fulfillment over the possibility of love.*

Sexual desire is natural, exciting, and something to cherish. Although forming one of the main bases for many relationships, sexual desire commonly leads to problems within relationships. Being attracted to someone is only the first step. A successful sexual relationship needs two people also to have compatible sexual desires. In cases where sexual desires do not match, education and communication can often bridge the gap. Sometimes, however, the gap is simply too wide. This chapter explores the multitude of issues that arise when sexual desire negatively affects relationships, and tries to explain what can be done to improve any problems and allow people to have more satisfying relationships.

Relationship Problems Caused by Sexual Desire

The most common sex-related problem we see with people is a mismatch in terms of the frequency or intensity of sexual desire within a couple. One person may want sex "somewhat" and "every so often," while their partner has desires every day and the desires are intense. Just because two people in a relationship have different intensities or frequencies of sexual desire does not mean necessarily that there is a pathology or an emotional/sexual problem. In fact, this is simply that people have mismatches in sexual desire. The mismatch or lack of fit could be situational (due to current circumstances, e.g. if one person is stressed at work) or could be a chronic issue to do with individual differences in sex drive or long-term issues (e.g. chronic stress). People can also have a mismatch in terms of what they find sexually arousing, irrespective of the environmental circumstances. Because sexual desire and attitudes vary massively between people, it is not surprising that a mismatch in sexual desires is a common issue in relationships. According to one study, 80 percent of couples experienced a mismatch in desire with their partner in the past month. There are also gender differences in attitudes toward sex.

Mismatch of Sexual Frequency/Intensity

Knowing that mismatches occur is half the battle. Without this awareness, couples may see a host of consequences. First, our partner's sexual desire has an effect on our self-esteem. Although we are all aware that this should not be the case, it is. We might want our partner to come home at the end of the day, have a hungry sexual look on their face, and look like they will explode with desire. This makes us feel wanted and attractive. Conversely, when our partner has little interest in sex, we might feel unwanted and unfortunately less worthwhile. Thus, problems can be felt from both sides of the couple. The higher-libido partner deals with repeated sexual rejection that may impact self-esteem, while the lower-libido partner may feel guilty and even overwhelmed by sexual pressure and feel like they are not living up to their partner's expectations.

Not feeling desired also raises issues about how to deal with the mismatch in sexual desire. If our partner lacks interest in us, do we say something? We do not want to be "desired" out of pity. In addition, we do not want to have someone tell us why they may not want sex with us. Perhaps they will mention my breath, that I am no good at sex, that I have gained weight, or that they no longer love me. Therefore, most of us simply wait to see if things will change. One problem with this approach is that we are harboring many feelings while we wait – fear, self-loathing, anger, and resentment. Left unaddressed, these pent-up negative feelings can build up. Another problem with this strategy is that things might not change. A person who has little sexual interest is unlikely to change as the current state of affairs may feel comfortable to them. Also, they are often unaware of how the other person may be interpreting the lack of sex. Perhaps they feel their partner is okay with it. Therefore, they are unlikely to mention or change anything.

The lack of interest from our partner may also lead to feelings or thoughts of infidelity. This can be from both directions. We may believe the person is cheating on us and feel distrustful or suspicious. This in turn may express itself as being unkind, terse, or nasty, all without any apparent provocation according to the other person's perspective. This could also lead us to consider infidelity: "Fine. If he is cheating on me, I might as well do the same." One can easily see how this could unravel the best of relationships.

We enter sexual relationships because we desire someone but also because we want to be desired. It is difficult to think we want someone more than they want us. This feels unequal and uncomfortable, both because we believe relationships should be equal but also because we fear that this means someone else could eventually mean more to our partner.

Talking about this issue is important, but equally important is how we discuss it. Nothing bothers a partner more, or kills sexual desire more quickly, than feeling like your partner is needy. Therefore, to keep asking a partner questions such as "Do you find me attractive? Are you more attracted to someone else?" or "Convince me that I mean as much to you as you do to me" may not be the best way to develop a successful relationship.

Addressing the Mismatch in Sexual Desire Frequency

Both parties need to accept that people have different levels of sexual desire, in terms of both frequency and intensity, either chronically or at various times in their lives. The sooner in a relationship that this is discussed and understood the better. Some differences are going to be chronic and then people need to negotiate whether or not they fit well together and where sexual desire is prioritized in their minds. Much like people differ in terms of their interest in health, travel, etc., they also differ in terms of sex. This difference may have greater or smaller significance in the context of a particular couple. Each person must be honest with themself about how important this issue is and then see it as similar to many other issues that a couple negotiates. If it cannot be worked out, then perhaps the couple should not be together.

In the case where sexual desire has changed for one party, then a different level of conversation needs to take place. The couple needs to discuss honestly and openly what has changed and what they can do about it. One person may feel that the other person has gained weight and they are not as attracted to them any longer. The person may feel petty bringing this up and the other person may feel hurt and unloved. How this is discussed is as important as what is said. This type of conversation is difficult for both parties but is necessary if the couple wants to have a healthy sexual relationship. Reaffirming love and commitment before discussing details may make this an easier conversation to have: "I love you, but this matters to me. Would you mind if we talked about it?" Health issues, financial issues, or one person's extended family issues may all be part of why the person is not interested in sex. Instead of hoping the partner will not notice or that it might go away, this needs to be discussed. If not, the other person may create a number of false explanations (see above).

In addition, if this lack of sexual desire is situational, the other person should know that the relationship may return to what it was originally. An example of this would be if one person is stressed because of financial pressures and so loses interest in sex; if the stressor is resolved with time, interest in sex is likely to return, so the problem may only be temporary. Explaining this can afford realistic hope for the other person and also makes them more helpful in understanding what the person may be going through and what they might need in terms of support. The partner becomes an ally instead of an outsider.

For both the chronic and the situational examples, however, couples should also remember that there are multiple types of intimacy, and that sensuality and eroticism may be important elements to continue, even when sexual desires do not match.

Mismatch of Sexual Activity

Couples may generally enjoy sex but not always see eye to eye on what they should do sexually. As in the example above, Stephen and his partner disagreed as to what they found stimulating sexually. This is a common issue. Men may want oral sex but their female partners may be uninterested in performing it, or vice versa. A gay man may want anal play but his partner may have no interest in doing this. Given the vast array of sexual activities that are possible, the examples of how couples may have a mismatch in the types of sexual acts they desire are endless.

One issue is that couples often fail to tell each other how important certain sexual topics are in their lives. So instead of mentioning these facts, they nudge their partner to do it, often using gestures or indications without being explicit, and when they are shot down, they do not bring it up again. This leads to a certain level of sexual frustration, which in turn can lead to underlying anger and resentment. In some people, it can also lead to infidelity as the person feels they need and deserve certain things sexually and they will find it outside the relationship.

A further issue is that the person with secretive desires can feel that their desires are less legitimate and, by extension, that they are as well. They may even feel disgusting or morally reprehensible for having such desires. For example, a man may feel like a "pervert" for desiring oral sex or when his wife expresses her disgust in performing it. Sexual desire is often associated with moral judgments. One person in the relationship may feel morally inferior when their desires are met with disgust or denial. It is important for both parties to recognize that desire takes many forms, and none of them is necessarily better or worse than others. The key in relationships is to find some compromise in sexual activities where both parties are fulfilled and do not feel their sexual desires are being judged.

Summary

It is rare that couples have perfectly matched sexual desires – desire for the same type and frequency of sex activities at the same times. Sex is a compromise. Any discrepancy in sexual desire can lead to relationship problems, but it does not have to be this way. We recommend that couples discuss any issues early on, rather than letting these fester beneath the surface. It helps to start these conversations by saying something positive, such as acknowledging that you love or really care for the person. Explain why discussing something is important to you. Choosing the right time (or best time) for such discussions is crucial: it is best to tackle difficult issues when both people are in a fresh frame of mind and have the time and mental space to do so, rather than when they are exhausted from a day of work or are worrying about going out in a few minutes. Lastly, we strongly recommend a few sessions of couples counseling for any couple – not just for couples who perceive they have major difficulties. Nothing is lost in doing so and, in our experience, many couples who try it find it very positive and useful to strengthen their relationship.

10 Sex and Digital Technology

David is a 55-year-old teacher who separated from his wife after living together for 15 years. Before the separation, David used pornography a few times a week and found it helped him maintain his sexual enthusiasm, including with his partner. Since the break-up, David has found himself using internet pornography for several hours per day, to which he masturbates several times a day. He has also found that he uses the Internet to gamble. He registered online for several gambling casinos because they offered free vouchers, but he used these and now finds his credit cards are at their limit, after losing a great deal of money to gambling. He feels like he has lost control over pornography use and gambling, and although they give him a "buzz," he is frustrated at not being able to control these activities and has started to experience thoughts that life might not be worth living. At the same time, he wonders whether these are addictions and whether they can be treated.

Julie is a business executive whose work involves a lot of travel. She has dated many women but finds it hard to establish a long-term relationship as she is away from home a lot. Julie has registered with several internet dating "apps" and finds that she spends many hours each day clicking "like" or "dislike" and also reading websites about online dating strategies and how to write

> *the perfect description. Julie is quite preoccupied with repeatedly checking for health-related information online, as she has developed some abdominal discomfort that has persisted for more than a year. Julie has seen her doctor several times and has had various investigations, which were normal. Julie does not feel reassured and repeatedly reads about bowel cancer and other possibilities on the Internet.*

The Internet has gone from not existing to being everywhere in just 30 years or so. It is hard to think of any other single societal change that has happened so quickly and with such a vast impact on the way people live across the globe. Digital technology has had a massive impact on our attitudes and behaviors relating to sex and desire. The term "cybersex" has emerged to describe a variety of sexual activities linked to technology use, from static pornography use to sexual interactions with others (whether for dating purposes or for more direct online sexual activities via webcams or chatrooms) to the use of sex toys linked to the Internet. While the Internet offers massive benefits to many in terms of being able to access resources rapidly and communicate with people from across the world, it is increasingly recognized that some people develop unhealthy or impairing habits in terms of their use of the Internet. As is often the case with topics related to sex, opinion tends to polarize. We do not take a moral stance with regard to these activities but rather seek to help people understand them, and to determine what the evidence shows, including potential positives and downsides that can be relevant depending on the person.

Internet Pornography

Multiple large-scale studies from across the world have shown that 70–95 percent of adults have used pornography at some point in their life (certainly the majority of men, and also the majority of women, although average rates of use are typically higher in men). While pornography use classically involved viewing "dirty magazines," the Internet now enables people to access diverse types of pornography almost immediately and at negligible financial cost. In one study of internet users, around 25 percent of women and 45 percent of men reported viewing internet pornography. Not surprisingly, rates of pornography use involving the Internet have gone up markedly with time, with the proliferation of internet connectivity and the number of websites catering to diverse sexual interests. There are many underlying reasons why people may use pornography online, and these differ among people. Studies show that common reasons people report for using pornography include obtaining sexual gratification/satisfaction, curiosity, emotional distraction, reducing stress, fantasy, alleviating boredom, and self-exploration. So, pornography use is not just about gratification in itself but may encompass multiple psychological drives.

Internet Pornography and Relationships

It might be tempting to assume that pornography use in relationships would be a bad thing: it might mean a person is fantasizing about other situations or people rather than the "real-life" partner. Internet pornography, some argue, can promote stereotypical perspectives about gender or sex, aggression, or unsafe sexual practices. As such, the content of some pornography is likely to be detrimental to an individual and their relationship. Certain forms of pornography of course are illegal or unhealthy because they transgress the bounds of accepted practice in a given country or involve exploitation, including of vulnerable people, or promote activities that are unhealthy.

Data show that use of pornography does not necessarily decrease substantially when people enter relationships. In fact, many people still continue to use pornography, including while they are in long-term stable relationships. Some of this internet pornography use relates to joint sexual activities, while other use continues to be self-masturbation separate from the relationship. As with many aspects of sexuality, the nature and extent of these activities is quite variable. One couple may enjoy mutual masturbation to pornography and find that this brings them emotionally closer together as well as providing sexual satisfaction. In another couple, if one person masturbates using pornography separate from their partner to the extent that they lose interest and ability to have sexual intercourse with their partner, that would be negative for the relationship. The pros and cons of pornography use in relationships are as diverse as the relationships themselves.

Only a few studies have examined the associations between internet pornography use and sexual well-being in couples. In one study, higher pornography use in women (whether on their own or with their partner) was associated with greater sexual well-being. However, the relationships between these variables were relatively small, suggesting that in fact the link is very complex and relates to a couple's individual circumstances. Some research suggests that using pornography could lead to men or women developing "idealized" images that are upsetting to their partner, whereas other studies have found that the use of pornography can facilitate sexual responsiveness in some couples. In terms of sexual satisfaction, the literature again has mixed results, but overall it seems that higher frequency of pornography use in men is associated with lower sexual satisfaction, with inconsistent findings in women. Much of this work is cross-sectional (i.e. all collected at the same time) and so we cannot say that one causes the other – we cannot say whether a higher frequency of pornography use leads to lower satisfaction, or whether lower sexual satisfaction leads to men seeking out pornography use, or whether another variable accounts for this statistical link.

Rates of sexual dysfunction in the general population appear to be increasing over time, especially in men under 40, although this could partly reflect men being more willing to acknowledge this in surveys. Often (but not always), erectile dysfunction in younger men is not due to a specific medical condition. Some authors have argued that this apparent increase in sexual dysfunction in younger men over time may partly be due to consequences of internet pornography use. Theoretically, the highly rewarding and fairly immediate satisfaction associated with internet pornography could result in some people finding that they cannot become sufficiently aroused by typical sexual activities with their partner in "real life" (as opposed to fantasies experienced through pornography or other online sex activities). The problem with these suggestions is that they are based on small numbers of case reports rather than on more rigorous scientific evidence. Overall, we think that these issues can occur in some cases, but feel that more research is needed to understand how common these problems are.

Internet Sex Addiction

While many people are able to use the Internet for sex in a way that suits them and is not harmful, it is increasingly recognized that some can develop excessive or "problematic" usage of the Internet that feels out of control and distressing, and leads to negative outcomes. There is now considerable evidence that so-called "problematic usage of the Internet" is associated with a variety of mental health problems. In a study of around 1,700 people, online pornography use showed a relatively strong link to problematic usage of the Internet, as did other online activities including general surfing, gaming, gambling, shopping, and social networking.

Whether we view problematic usage of internet pornography as an "addiction" is a matter of perspective. It is not currently considered to be a recognized psychiatric condition. At the same time, it is quite clear that some people lose control over their internet pornography use and that this has negative consequences and fulfills many of the classic criteria for addiction, such as difficulty cutting back on the behavior, persisting behavior despite negative effects on life, loss of control over the behavior, and concealing the activities from others. In Chapter 3, we saw that certain behaviors can activate the brain's ancient reward pathways, triggering the release of chemicals such as dopamine. We know from neuroimaging research that brains of people with compulsive sexual behavior show a stronger response to viewing pornography than people without it – and there is no reason to believe that viewing pornography over the Internet would be any different. Depending on exactly how it is defined, data show that around 1–4 percent of the population experience problematic internet pornography use. Just because pornography use is frequent in a person, however, does not mean it is necessarily problematic. In a large study of internet users, around 20 percent of the sample fitted best into a category that had a high frequency of pornography use but did not have "problematic" pornography use. Approximately 10 percent of the sample had both high-frequency pornography use and some degree of problematic use. This higher rate of 10 percent, compared with the population rate of 1–4 percent quoted above, probably reflects the different ways of defining "problematic" use.

Internet Pornography, Sex, and Younger People

Viewing of internet pornography by younger people has been a focus of particular concern. Given that the Internet (e.g. social media, apps, communication tools) is a major part of many young people's lives, exposure to pornography is common. Some young people may view pornography intentionally, whereas others may be exposed to pornography without intending to view it due to "pop-ups" and advertisements, or from being forwarded sexually explicit pornography from others. In surveys, 25–65 percent of adolescents reported having viewed pornography, but young people reported that in most cases this involved unintentional viewing. However, of those who had viewed pornography, more than half reported viewing it weekly. This suggests a range of frequency of use but also perhaps underreporting of intentional use, due to shame or the stigmatized nature of sexual activities at a time when younger people are developing a sexual identity and awakening.

An important concern that has been widely raised is the prospect that by being exposed to internet pornography involving unrealistic expectations of sexual acts, body images, and relationships, young people in particular may develop maladaptive perspectives on what real-world sexual relationships might involve, particularly if internet pornography is the main form of sexual stimulus shaping and sculpting their developing psychosexual brains. For example, these expectations could lead to young people and their partners being pressured into particular sexual activities or early sexual activities that they otherwise would eschew. Young people might consider sex (or particular sex acts) to be integral to relationships in people of their age, whereas in reality, sex (or particular sex acts) may be uncommon in the given age group. For some, online pornography could warp their perspectives of peer-group and wider cultural norms.

Because online platforms are not subject to people seeing each other in natural environments where they may know each other personally, this can render young people especially vulnerable to exploitation and grooming. Young people may receive unwanted communications (from people their age but also from adults) such as unwanted sexual advances, intrusion of their privacy, and/or attempts at manipulation. At the same time, studies show that many young people are quite well informed of online risks and know how to block or report inappropriate contacts.

Internet Dating Apps

Internet websites and applications are now widely used to help people find partners, whether for sexual liaisons or longer-term sexual relationships. According to Business of Apps, 270 million people across the world used dating apps in 2020, and this is increasing at a steady rate. Currently, the most commonly used app is Tinder, but there are a multitude of apps that purport to have advantages over others, or to be useful for people wanting specific types of relationship. For example, there are apps targeting those looking for long-term partners rather than hook-ups, apps for people with different sexual orientations, and apps for people from different cultural backgrounds.

Roughly 10 percent of people use dating apps, depending on the sample being surveyed – some surveys report much higher levels. Apps can offer potential advantages over conventional approaches of meeting people such as being less intimidating, enabling more efficient inter-actions, and enabling access to a greater diversity and num-bers of potential partners. In theory, data algorithms could make success more likely than just meeting people haphaz-ardly through real-life social networks, but the evidence for this is not clear. The majority of dating app users say that their main aim is not to have sex but rather for other motivations, such as looking for new friends or long-term partners, although men on average are more likely than women to use apps for sex as a primary motivation.

Due to their relative newness, research on whether dating apps have associations with mental health and well-being is fairly limited. In a review of around 70 studies, similar proportions of men and women were found to be using dating apps in their lives. People of many different ages reported using dating apps, from adolescents through to older people, but their usage seems most common in those aged 24–30 years. Dating apps seem to be more com-monly used, on average, in individuals who have minority sexual orientations, perhaps especially those in cultures and locations where meeting partners is particularly difficult (e.g. due to the physical rarity of being able to meet new people, or where minority perspectives are stigmatized in the local community). Overall, 10–30 percent of people who use dating apps report having a partner already, so they are not used only by single people. Certain personality traits are linked to using dating apps, especially open-mindedness.

Are apps successful in enabling people to meet and share sexual experiences? Measuring this is difficult because people who find them unsuccessful are arguably less likely to take part in a survey asking about success. In addition, perhaps using apps excessively means people may be less likely to seek out partners through more conventional means. We also have to bear in mind that it is in the interests of the app industry to report higher levels of success than may actually be the case. Overall, data suggest that around 25–35 percent of users find a romantic partner via dating apps, and that 15–50 percent of dating app users report having casual sex with at least one person they met through a dating app.

Despite the potential advantages of dating apps, their use also raises a number of issues, particularly for more vulnerable people. We stress that we take a neutral view: we cannot say that dating apps are intrinsically good or bad for self-esteem or mental health. It depends on the person and context. But it is important to highlight not only the advantages but also the downsides that may occur.

Dating apps can have a negative effect on well-being and mental health in some people. Perhaps not surprisingly, the link between self-esteem and dating app use is inconsistent. Some people may have high self-esteem and use the app confidently as a means of meeting others. For others, low self-esteem may mean that dating apps offer new opportunities to meet people using a mechanism that feels more comfortable than going up to someone in a bar, or asking someone out on a date face to face, which could improve self-esteem. At the same time, some apps are quite harsh and judgmental: if someone obtains large numbers of "not likes" through a dating app, or finds that they do not meet a partner despite extensive efforts, this could exacerbate low self-esteem and contribute to mental health difficulties.

For some individuals, dating apps can engender deceit or put people into vulnerable situations. Potential partners are met out of context of a usual social network, and a usual social network may offer protection against being taken advantage of, or coming into contact with someone who is potentially violent. As noted, a significant proportion of people using dating apps are already in long-term relationships, so they can offer an efficient channel for deceiving partners, but in some cases partners may be aware of app use and even support it (e.g. to have threesomes, or having agreed open relationships).

In a study that focused on "swipe-based" apps, where users indicate they like or dislike suggested individuals, more people reported a positive impact of app use on self-esteem than a negative impact. However, app use was associated with higher levels of distress, low mood, and anxiety. So it seems users may view apps as a good thing, but their use can have negative associations nonetheless. As is common for cross-sectional studies, this research cannot say whether the link between variables is causal or not – i.e. whether app use leads to problems, or whether people with lower mood are more likely to start using apps, perhaps even to help with the low mood. It is also unclear how the pros and cons of dating apps compare with very similar positive and negatives attributes of in-person dating.

Another consideration is that a proportion of people using dating apps excessively have a wider problem referred to as "problematic usage of the Internet," meaning they use the Internet in a harmful way for a variety of activities, including but not limited to sex and dating. Problematic internet usage can lead to people spending large amounts of time on apps but also engaging in other online activities, not only those relating to sex. This problematic usage can also negatively affect life in other ways, due to loss of control, escalating use over time, and neglect of other areas of life. In a large study of Tinder users, participants were classified into groups using a statistical modeling approach: 25 percent of the sample had problematic use, which was associated with being more impulsive but with reasonable self-esteem, while 30 percent of the sample had some degree of problematic use but linked more to depression and low self-esteem. Overall, it seemed that about half of the sample had some degree of problematic internet use linked to dating apps, but again it cannot be concluded that one necessarily causes the other.

Given that dating apps can lead to sex, and sex can lead to sexually transmitted diseases or early pregnancy, there are also public health and personal health considerations. In a survey, unprotected sex was associated with the use of dating apps, as well as earlier age at first sexual intercourse and older age, plus smoking and alcohol use. The authors also reported that those people using dating apps were less likely than others to have used a condom in their most recent sexual encounter.

Practical Advice on Safe Internet Sex and Dating

As we have seen, the Internet offers potential advantages for sex but also a number of risks and potential disadvantages. A primary consideration is that the Internet may seem anonymous, but it stores information, potentially forever. It is not uncommon for employers to search the Internet, including social media, for potential new staff, and anyone can search for information about you online. Be careful about putting sensitive information in a public forum, or in a forum that is just a few steps removed from being public, such as social media. Personal information to be cautious about exposing can include clues on where you live, any travel plans (e.g. saying when you are away from home), or any other sensitive information. We find that a suitably cautious approach is to ask yourself, "If this information potentially became available to literally anybody on the Internet, would I feel comfortable with that?" The safe-guards for social media and many related apps, including dating apps, are not stringent. Even if the software does have data-protection safeguards, sometimes personal data can be leaked due to hackers or even faulty code, or by companies selling information onward to other companies. Be aware also that you may share information with people you trust, but those people may then share that information with others – either deliberately or unintentionally.

For parents, sitting down with your children to discuss safe use of the Internet is valuable, as this may not be taught at schools. Often the young person might be extremely educated about safe online use – even more so than their parents – but having a dialog open about the topic is healthy, and everyone may learn from each other. Also consider safeguards – many internet providers allow parents to set safety features such as blocking dangerous or inappropriate material. Be aware, though, that this does not override the need to have an open two-way discussion with your children: young people are smart and can often bypass these restrictions. Also, they can access the Internet from many places, not only the home, so home safeguards can only go so far in protecting the young person. In terms of practical tips for internet use in general, a European group of experts have developed a free book, *Learning to Deal with Problematic Usage of the Internet* (see Selected Literature and Further Reading for this chapter), that includes practical strategies on using the Internet safely, including top tips for parents.

For pornography use in the context of relationships, if this is something you do privately and you feel it does not impact the relationship, then it is probably OK to carry on and not discuss it. However, if you feel your use of pornography could be affecting your relationship (e.g. you no longer have any sex drive with your partner, or find your pornography use becoming excessive or hard to control), then it is worth discussing, as is also the case if your partner has mentioned it. Such discussions can be tricky because we all have preconceptions about pornography and what is acceptable, much of which reflects our upbringing (parenting) as well as the norms of networks we grew up around. Some people enjoy using pornography during sex with their partners, and having an open discussion about sex and what each person likes during sex, while initially uncomfortable, is often a good thing in the longer term for a relationship.

For dating through the Internet or using digital apps, we have several suggestions. First, if you are thinking about using a dating app, do some research into what app(s) might be best for you: some are more focused on people wanting long-term relationships, whereas others are more about casual sex. Read the privacy documents the app provider has, and read reviews from people who have used these apps, by searching on the Internet (look beyond reviews on the app's own website, as often these are deliberately spun to be positive, with negative reviews removed, often in return for a reward). Next, think carefully about what images and written information you put on your dating profile or share with others. Again, would you be comfortable if this information found its way into the public domain so everyone could see it, which is basically the worst-case scenario but can happen. If not, are you confident the company providing the app has really stringent data safeguards in place and encryption? Also, avoid sharing material that means a person could pinpoint where you live, or know a lot about your normal routine, or learn about your banking information or the services you use, as well as when you might tend to be at work or otherwise away from home. Be wary if you come across someone online who is keen to avoid using the dating platform (e.g. shifting to another means of communication before you have met them face to face), asks personally sensitive information, or makes requests for gift cards or anything of value. This may seem obvious, but, scams are often so sophisticated now that many extremely smart and knowledgeable people have been fooled out of substantial amounts of money and personally sensitive information online, or put into unwanted and potentially dangerous scenarios. Remember, too, that unless you are using a reputable app that conducts rigorous background checks, the details someone provides online may be nothing to do with them: they may use someone else's photo, life, or even completely fictitious information.

Prior to going on an actual date with someone you have met over the Internet or through an app, take your time to consider what you are comfortable with and where is a safe place to meet, as well as what you can do if something goes wrong. It is sensible to have dates in a public location such as a café with plenty of people around, and to have a plan in mind for an excuse if for any reason you feel uncomfortable and wish to leave early (e.g. you could have a plan in advance to say you need to leave for a work meeting or because you are meeting a friend). If you think of an "escape plan" in advance, it will be easier to use it in the moment, rather than trying to come up with an excuse spontaneously. Before going on a date, ensure your telephone is fully charged (in case you need to call anyone, e.g. if you are feeling in a difficult situation) and tell a friend where you are going and agree to text them afterwards to tell them you are OK, and what time they should hear from you. You could even suggest a friend goes along with you on a first date: ask the person you are due to meet if they would be happy for a friend to come along, even if the friend sits separately. If they are a reputable person, they would not have a reason to object to this, especially in the very early stages of meeting someone for the first time.

Summary

This chapter has considered the important and varied ways the Internet now plays a role in sex and relationships – for better and for worse. It is evident that the benefits as well as the downsides or risks of using the Internet for sex-related activities are very varied, depending on the context and individual. We cannot generalize and say, for example, that pornography is intrinsically good or bad for relationships. In the case of David in the case vignette, his online pornography use shifted over time, from being positive to becoming out of control and impairing, and he found it rewarding like gambling. In the case of Julie, she initially used the Internet for practical and beneficial purposes, using a dating app, and searching out initial medical information about symptoms she was experiencing to alleviate anxiety. But over time, she found herself spending inordinate amounts of time using the Internet to the extent that she found it negatively affecting her well-being and quality of life, and reinforcing her anxieties.

The secret is to make the Internet work best– and safely – for you and those around you by considering the benefits and risks of, for example, online dating or viewing online pornography, and to watch out for signs of problematic usage of the Internet (i.e. excessive use that leads to negative outcomes). Also consider that the way we engage with the Internet and technology is not static, and the benefits and risks for us can change over time, as in the case vignettes. We recommend that couples discuss their use of online technology for sex with each other. Parents can promote safe online use for their children through two-way discussions and use of appropriate safeguards.

11   Diverse Aspects of Sex

Samantha is a 35-year-old woman who identifies as bisexual and has been married for 2 years to her female partner. Prior to this, Samantha was married to a man for 4 years. She has two children who live with her and her female partner. During her first marriage, Samantha realized that she was not exclusively heterosexual and in fact had an affair with her current partner. This led to the dissolution of her first marriage. Since that time, Samantha has struggled with feelings of low self-esteem, often unsure if she was or is currently "living a lie" as she has never really been comfortable with herself sexually. She enjoys sex with her female partner but misses aspects of sex with her ex-husband. In addition, she often feels that she "does not know who she is" when having sex. These feelings of confusion have led her to drink alcohol more in the evening prior to having sex as she believes it calms her down and makes having sex more relaxed. To compound the issues further, Samantha has recently felt an attraction to a male coworker. She fantasizes about him at times when having sex with her partner. Samantha worries that these feelings and confusion about sexual desire could mean the end of her second marriage.

Todd is a 25-year-old male and works full-time. Todd never dated during his college years and, although he knew he was gay, he never acted on these feelings because of fears

> *of acquiring sexually transmitted diseases and from*
> *embarrassment about the fact that he never knew exactly*
> *what one does when having gay sex or how to do it well.*
> *While working, Todd began having sexual feelings for*
> *a coworker who was about 15 years his senior. Todd wanted*
> *to ask him out but felt intimidated because he was out of*
> *shape, whereas his senior coworker was very healthy. He*
> *feared that gay men only wanted well-built men as part-*
> *ners. In addition, Todd worried that perhaps this man*
> *might have a sexually transmitted disease, given that he*
> *has been dating men for many years.*

When speaking of sexual desire, we often assume incorrectly that everyone has the same issues and that the same solutions are appropriate for all groups. Researchers have noted that cross-cultural attempts to study sexuality have often been limited by focusing only on "marriage" and "family," with other topics being taboo or just not within the cultural framework of the people conducting the research. Another issue is that much research on sexuality has been limited to a Western focus, and we certainly acknowledge these limitations for the purposes of the current book. Collectively, these issues hinder our understanding of minority groups and diversity. Discrimination, marginalization, and violence against minorities – including LGBTQ people – occur every-where in the world, albeit to varying degrees. Political and other community leaders may promote initiatives against sexual desire in the LGBTQ community as means of "safe-guarding morality and social order." LGBTQ individuals are attributed all sorts of negative qualities connected to their sexual orientation, and this may lead to poor self-esteem and a host of other issues regarding their sexual desire. Thus, the LGBTQ community may have unique issues that need to be addressed. The topic of diversity and sex cannot be completely covered by a single chapter in a book and most likely deserves several books on its own. Having said that, our aim in this chapter is to present a select sample of topics that pertain to the LGBTQ community and by doing so help to inform a broader understanding of sexual desire and diversity.

Much of this chapter reports findings on gay men and lesbians, as this is where the research has primarily been focused. What about the sexual desires of individuals who identify as bisexual? A large number of people experience some degree of fluidity in their sexual and romantic attractions, being drawn to the same gender at one point in their life and the opposite gender at another. There is also extensive evidence that sexuality can alter over time in a given individual. Another consideration is that people can experience same-sex attraction while having a heterosexual identity. In research across several countries, 16–21 percent of men and 17–19 percent of women reported either same-sex behavior or same-sex attraction, despite identifying as heterosexual.

Even with these numbers, bisexuality has often been maligned, both by anti-LGBTQ forces who believe bisexuals are necessarily nonmonogamous, and by some gays and lesbians who consider bisexuality merely a stage on the way to a gay or lesbian identity – or perhaps denial of such an identity. Bisexual individuals face unique challenges and varied forms of discrimination and erasure.

While bisexuals face many of the same hardships that gays and lesbians encounter, they often face the additional burden of discrimination by both heterosexuals and homosexuals. Some people even refuse to believe that bisexuality exists. Bisexuals are relatively invisible because most people have a tendency to presume that all individuals are either gay or straight, depending on the gender of their current partner. Bisexuals are also less likely than their gay and lesbian peers to make their underlying status public.

Biology of LGBTQ Desire

Many of those who oppose LGBTQ equality dismiss the biological basis of sexual orientation and promote other theories regarding the development of an LGBTQ orientation. Some argue that gay male desire develops as a result of certain types of parenting such as the presence of an overly involved mother and/or absent father. There is no evidence to suggest that how people parent their children has any direct involvement in the type of sexual orientation a child subsequently develops. Recent research suggests that genetics and hormonal influences in the uterus may result in an LGBTQ orientation.

Although grouped together under the label of LGBTQ, there may be significant differences among the various groups. In fact, some researchers have also concluded that there are biological bases for transgender identity (e.g. neuroanatomical differences, such as brain gray- and white-matter studies, and steroid hormone genetics, such as genes associated with sex hormone receptors) and they appear different from the nascent biological findings in gay men and lesbians.

Differences in Sexual Desire Based on Sexual Orientation

There is a general social perception of gay men being hypersexual. In reality, they are no more interested in sex than heterosexual individuals. Because they are pursuing other men, gay men may be more successful than their heterosexual counterparts. There has been suggestion that the only difference in frequency of sex among gay men compared with heterosexual men is perhaps contingent upon gender differences. The desire of the two groups does not differ but the actual sexual behavior might. In fact, a large international study found that gay and bisexual men were somewhat lower in sex drive than heterosexual men, whereas bisexual women were higher in sex drive than heterosexual and lesbian women.

Although contrary to the data, the perception of gay as hypersexual places a certain amount of pressure on gay men, particularly in relationships. Gay male couples feel a lot of pressure to remain sexually exciting. Gay men may feel inadequate if they are not hypersexual, and they may blame themselves for problems in the relationship. Education around this topic can reduce this sense of self-flagellation and allow gay men to realize that their sexual desires will wax and wane depending upon what is going on in their lives, in the relationship, and in their health.

Issues in LGBTQ Sexual Relationships

There are often unique issues with regard to LGBTQ relationships. One issue unique to LGBTQ individuals is the concept of "coming out." One person in a homosexual couple may be out to family, friends, and work colleagues, while the other is not. This may result in frustration for both parties. Being able to make peace with one's identity and world can bring a couple closer.

Another issue among LGBTQ couples is that of sexual satisfaction. Sexual satisfaction in a relationship has a direct correlation with overall relationship satisfaction. Sexual desire and sexual frequency do not stem from the same domains: sexual desire characterizes an underlying aspect of sexual motivation and is associated with romantic feelings, while actual sexual activity and intercourse are associated with the development and advancement of a given relationship. Thus, together, sexual desire and sexual frequency can successfully predict the stability of a relationship.

Low sexual desire discrepancies (low sexual desire and low sexual frequency) are common among lesbian couples, similar to heterosexual women in a relationship with a man. The sexual frequency between lesbian couples has been reported as less frequent in comparison with gay male, heterosexual, married, and unmarried couples. One study looking at 1,500 lesbian women who were in relationships found low levels of sexual contact, suggesting relatively low sexual desire.

Studies show that lesbians are particularly prone to internalizing negative homophobic societal attitudes, which has detrimental effects on their self-esteem and identity. It has been proposed that lesbians may show a tendency to use defenses in an attempt to deny their homosexuality in a homophobic society. Lesbians may therefore manifest strong emotional connections to their partners but repress any sexual desires due to an unconscious internalization of society's homophobic attitudes, which ultimately manifests in a reduced sexual desire and sexual intercourse frequency.

Gay male couples in long-term relationships often complain that they have not been sexual for long periods of time, sometimes years. They may tell us that they have agreed to get sex outside their relationship, or they are only sexual with each other when it involves a third man. These men question whether they are really right for each other, if they are not able to keep sex alive between just the two of them. It is not only gay couples for whom sexual activity tapers off after the initial honeymoon period. For both gay and straight individuals, sexual excitement typically wanes after the first 2 or 3 years. To bring passion and sex back into your relationship, you have to want to do it and realize that it takes work.

Some approaches to bringing sex back into a relationship are the same for both LGBTQ and non-LGBTQ couples, for example the importance of setting time aside for intimacy. Most couples – gay and straight – insist that they should not have to plan for sex, which should come naturally and spontaneously the way it did in the beginning of their relationship. However, planning can help you anticipate being together, making sex more exciting.

Similarly, couples should try to focus on some detail they find attractive about their partner. People change over time, they put on weight, lose some hair, and no longer seem as sexy – or no longer seem sexy in the same way. Couples need to learn to focus on the aspects of the person they do like and the things that arouse them. Additionally, couples may also find it useful to reconnect on an intimate level without sex. Take a bath or shower together or lie naked beside each other. Gay couples not having sex for long periods of time can now come out of the closet of shame and lonely isolation, knowing that their worry is more common than generally talked about.

Issues in transgender relationships may be more complex. Partners of transgender people may or may not have sexual orientations that are congruent with their partner's gender. For example, a male-to-female (MTF) person who was married to a woman throughout her transition may remain married. Post-transition, the MTF person may now identify as lesbian, while the MTF's wife may still identify as heterosexual. Such relationship issues may require ongoing negotiations and compromises about what is important in a relationship and how best to navigate these changes.

LGBTQ Couples and Open Relationships

Research shows that many gay couples open their relationships after 5–7 years together. In fact, studies show that more than 40 percent of gay men had an agreement that sex outside the relationship was permissible, while less than 5 percent of heterosexual and lesbian couples reported the same. These couples can communicate and have agreements with each other so that both know that neither one is cheating or doing anything in secret. This frank openness may help partners to reactivate sexual desire in one another. In fact, some research suggests that this clear and open communication about desire also builds a stronger bond in a relationship. This may be the reason that some studies of open relationships in gay men have found that nonmonogamous couples can actually be closer than their more faithful monogamous counterparts.

Other Issues with LGBTQ Individuals

Despite rapidly growing cultural acceptance of diverse sexual and romantic orientations and gender identifications, oppression, discrimination, and marginalization of LGBTQ people persists. Coping with discrimination and oppression, coming out to one's family, and sorting out an "authentic" sense of self in the face of social expectations and pressures (e.g. the case of Samantha above) can lead to higher levels of depression, anxiety, substance use, suicide, and other mental health concerns for LGBTQ people.

Research shows that youth who identify as LGBTQ are at an increased risk of suicidal ideation (i.e. suicidal thoughts) and self-harm, particularly when they also experience discrimination based on their sexual or gender identity. According to research, students who identified as LGBTQ were almost 10 times as likely to have experienced bullying and victimization at school and more than twice as likely to have considered suicide as their heterosexual, nontransgender classmates within the previous year.

Discrimination may take several forms, including social rejection, verbal and physical bullying, and sexual assault, and repeated episodes will likely lead to chronic stress and diminished mental health. Perceived discrimination, or the expectation of discrimination, may also lead to worse mental health. LGBTQ adults, too, may be subject to similar forms of harassment, as well as discrimination with regard to housing, employment, education, and basic human rights.

Anxiety and confusion over sexual orientation are common in LGBTQ individuals, as in the case of Samantha. Many LGBTQ individuals report initial confusion about their true orientation. This may particularly be the case where the person identifies as being bisexual. This confusion can lead to anxiety about the stability of a relationship and the person's ability to commit to someone in a relationship. When one orientation is more socially acceptable, this may lead to greater anxiety, guilt, and internalized homophobia (negative internalized feelings about being LGBTQ).

When the believed cause for sexual desire discrepancy is thought to be a form of internalized homophobia, it is often useful to examine the individual's feelings toward being homosexual, for example by asking questions such as: "How do you feel about being lesbian?", "Have you ever felt suicidal as a result of your homosexuality?", or "In what way do you think homosexual people are different from hetero-sexual people?" Support may consist of referrals to LGBTQ social and education groups for exposure to positive role models.

Influence of HIV on LGBTQ Sexual Desire

LGBTQ issues, particularly those of gay and bisexual men and transgender people, have long been associated with and to some extent defined by the HIV/AIDS epidemic. In terms of the influence of HIV on sexual desire, there are both the psychological aspects of getting the illness and the actual health aspects of being HIV positive.

The psychological approach to HIV/AIDS among LGBTQ individuals has been complex and has changed over time. Both "prevention fatigue" (difficulty maintaining safer-sex habits) and disinhibition (underestimating the consequences of HIV infection) are at play when under-standing sexual desire in the LGBTQ community. Deciding to follow safer-sex practices requires information, motivation, and time. Eventually the person may slip into episodes of unsafe behavior. Paradoxically, negative tests can reinforce the idea that safer sex is not needed.

Additionally, the success of anti-HIV medications in reducing progression to AIDS, prolonging life, and restor-ing quality of life for people with HIV has reduced fear of the virus. A common perception is that treatment will take care of an infection if it were to occur, and many people are unaware that progression to AIDS and development of HIV resistance still occur, and that treatment comes with significant side effects and demands strict adherence. Viral load testing is also partially to blame for the more relaxed attitude toward HIV. "Undetectable" levels of HIV can wrongly be taken as a license to have unprotected sex based on the assumption that, when undetectable, there is a very low risk of the virus being transmitted. Efforts to counter this misinformation have achieved varying levels of success.

Overall, it appears that as one group adopts safer-sex practices, another comes along and engages in risky behaviors. While new cases in adolescent and younger adults are still growing, there are fewer new HIV cases among those aged 25–44, the generation exposed to prevention measures in the last decade. A similar drop occurred among African-Americans. The current focus of the US Centers for Disease Control and Prevention (CDC) prevention efforts is "prevention for positives," encouraging people with HIV to practice safer sex. The emphasis is now on HIV testing, as the CDC has found that the majority of new sexually transmitted infections involve people unaware of their HIV status.

Infection with HIV/AIDS has become a chronic medical condition rather than a terminal diagnosis for most HIV-positive individuals in the developed world. The rate of sexual problems (e.g. low sexual desire, erectile dysfunction) in HIV-positive individuals (including HIV-positive men who have sex with men) has been reported to exceed the baseline incidence in the general population. Furthermore, most studies have reported that advanced HIV infection and AIDS portend a greater risk of sexual concerns and a decline in sexuality activity relative to less advanced HIV infection. This is not only an important quality-of-life issue but may also have relevance to public health because sexual problems may predispose some individuals to unsafe sexual practices (e.g. failure to use condoms). In studies that have included an HIV-negative group, sexual problems in HIV-positive adults (i.e. decreased sexual desire and erectile dysfunction) have been associated with advanced age, a lower CD4 count, and depression.

A number of pathophysiological disturbances probably contribute to sexual dysfunction in HIV disease, and the relative importance of different etiologies likely varies with stage of illness, disease complication, therapeutic intervention, age, and risk-factor group. To date, androgen deficiency is the most widely cited cause of sexual dysfunction in HIV-positive men. Specifically, low testosterone levels have been found in 6 percent of men with asymptomatic HIV infection and 50 percent men with AIDS. Individuals with asymptomatic disease were found to have significantly higher mean levels of testosterone than individuals with symptomatic HIV infection or AIDS.

Aging, Sexual Desire, and the LGBTQ Community

In our culture, the stigma against growing older is known as "ageism." Studies have shown that among older adults, approximately 80 percent have experienced at least one form of ageism in their day-to-day lives. According to the WHO, older adults who internalize negative attitudes about aging may live 7.5 years less than those with positive attitudes.

This stigma is pronounced in the gay community, given its emphasis on youth and physical beauty. For men who have bought into the conventional standards of gay attractiveness, aging can be terrifying. One study found that two-thirds of gay men felt that aging was more difficult due to the perception that gay men value youth.

LGBTQ people, like increasing numbers of persons in the general population, however, are shifting their views of aging toward seeing it as potentially full and rich. They do not deny the reality of old age and death, but this new attitude allows many mature men to have a zestful sexual life.

Although the stresses of aging experienced by LGBTQ individuals are similar to those of heterosexuals, older LGBTQ adults face issues of a stigmatized sexual orientation, invisibility, negative stereotypes, and discrimination regarding aging. For example, prior to the mid-1970s, the social stereotype of an older gay man was that he no longer goes to bars because he has lost his physical attractiveness and his sexual appeal to the young men he craves. He is oversexed, but his sex life is very unsatisfactory. He has been unable to form a lasting relationship with a sexual partner, and he is seldom sexually active anymore. When he does have sex, it is usually in a public arena. He has disengaged from the gay world and his acquaintances in it. In short, his life is composed of little intimacy and little sex. Contrary to this view, research has shown that the sex life of the older gay man is, characteristically, quite satisfactory, with desired sexual contact and intimacy with adult men, especially those near his own age, continued sexual contacts, long-term relationships, and involvement in the gay community. In fact, the pattern of sexual activity a man had in his youth tends to persist as he ages. In several surveys, as many as three-quarters of older gay men reported being happy with their sexual life. In some studies, over half of these men reported having sex at least once a week with a partner, and this was in addition to masturbating.

Lesbians may have a different course of aging compared with gay men. Among the most significant biological changes that women deal with as they age is menopause. Although menopause often comes with substantial physical changes, research has shown that 75 percent of lesbians reported that their sex lives were as good as before or more enjoyable after menopause. Some of the positive sexual changes in their lives since menopause included increased orgasms, increased sexual frequency, greater self-acceptance, and greater freedom.

Changes with the body as we age may have a less negative influence among lesbians. Lesbians may be less vulnerable than heterosexual peers to cultural attitudes that only youthful bodies are beautiful and sexually attractive. Because lesbians are not in sexual relationships with men, the importance of standard norms about physical appearance may be lessened. Lesbians' conception of physical attractiveness tends to emphasize such functional qualities as agility, stamina, and strength rather than characteristics conventionally valued in women by heterosexual men. Whether a lesbian rated her partner as physically beautiful or not did not affect her own sexual fulfillment, her happiness, or her belief that the relationship will last.

Summary

This chapter has described many facets of sexual behavior in the LGBTQ community. To better summarize the main points, we would like to return to the cases of Samantha and Todd. These cases show that many variables can influence the sexual identity and sexual desires of individuals within the LGBTQ community. Sexuality may, to some extent, be fluid, and coming out and the psychological fears of LGBTQ identity may influence sexual desires. LGBTQ individuals have different social and personal experiences that they navigate as part of their sexual desires.

12   Sex and Pandemics

Brian is a 37-year-old male, who is single and has been working from home during the COVID-19 pandemic. Although he was used to going out to meet women on the weekends, he essentially stopped doing so during the pandemic. Instead, Brian reports that he began using pornography as a substitute, and masturbating. Over time, however, Brian found that he was masturbating multiple times some days, and now that restrictions have loosened, he prefers to stay home and masturbate to pornography instead of spending time with friends or trying to date.

Deidre is a 42-year-old married women with no children. During the COVID-19 pandemic, her husband lost his job and she has become the sole source of financial support for the two of them. She works virtually from home and is doing longer hours than she ever worked when going to the office. She is stressed most days, has poor sleep, and has been eating unhealthy foods and has gained quite a bit of weight. She has no interest in sex and has a poor body image. Her husband initiates sexual contact every few days, but she is uninterested. Because of this, the couple has grown apart with few conversations, despite them both being home almost every day.

For the past 2 years approximately (at the time of writing), the world has been embroiled in a pandemic the likes of which has not been seen for quite some time. We have all heard the reports that the recent pandemic has increased rates of stress, anxiety, and depression in many people. Financial difficulties have also been commonplace. What effects, if any, has the pandemic had on people and their sex lives or desires?

Single during a Pandemic

In an effort to slow the spread of the COVID-19 pandemic, governments around the world began implementing restrictions on social contact. These restrictions resulted in significant changes in our work and leisure lives, including our sexual lives. For those living alone, the lockdowns were essentially mandating celibacy for most people. In fact, public health officials have described COVID-19 as similar to any other infectious disease that is associated with sexual activity. Sexual intimacy appears to be a high-risk situation for the transmission of COVID with simple kissing as a clear type of contact through which it can be transmitted. A recent survey asked if people would require their partner to submit to a COVID-19 test before becoming intimate, and slightly more than 40 percent said they would. In addition, 71 percent said that a person's vaccination status plays a major role in whether they would date them. This in turn resulted in some dating apps altering their platforms to allow users to narrow their search by identifying potential matches based on COVID-19 vaccination status. One popular app reported that people who indicated they were vaccinated against

COVID-19 received 14 percent more matches than those who were unvaccinated.

With greater COVID-19 restrictions, sexual behavior appears to have changed, at least to some degree. Some of the changes were an increase in the use of online pornography and an increase in erotic posts on social media. The extent of increase in pornography appeared related to the degree of lockdown and social isolation. Because having consensual sex with other people presented new health risks, one study found that approximately 70 percent of single adults reported reducing their number of sex partners as a result of the pandemic.

Although there was no evidence for a change in relationship satisfaction in general terms, both men and women reported a small decrease in sexual pleasure, and women reported a small decrease in sexual desire, during the pandemic. The sexual behaviors with greatest reduction were casual sex, hook-ups, and number of partners, and the most diminished aspect of sexual functioning was sexual enjoyment. Depression symptoms, relationship status, and perceived importance of social distancing emerged as predictors of these reductions.

As one would expect, not everyone has responded to the pandemic in the same fashion. An online survey of 1,559 adults found that although approximately 50 percent reported a decline in their sex life, 20 percent reported expanding their sexual repertoire by incorporating new activities. Common additions included sexting, trying new sexual positions, and sharing sexual fantasies. Being younger, living alone, and feeling stressed and lonely were linked to trying new things.

Participants making new additions were three times more likely to report improvements in their sex life.

Couples and the Pandemic

The COVID-19 pandemic appears to have had some effects on couples as well. Multiple variables – children being taught at home, parents having to change their work schedule to accommodate children being home, living in close quarters day in and day out, and financial stresses of people losing their jobs – have all been associated with both reduced partnered bonding behaviors (for example, cuddling, holding hands) as well as reduced partnered sexual behaviors.

Interestingly, for all of the stress secondary to COVID-19 as well as the change in sexual behaviors, the divorce rate has actually gone down during the pandemic. Perhaps due to the trauma associated with a pandemic, there has been an increase in commitment and gratitude in marriages. Fewer people have entered marriage since the pandemic, but there has been more stability in those who are married. Similarly, although there has been increased and different stressors due to children during the pandemic, research demonstrates that married people with children have been happier than childless married couples.

COVID-19 and Sexually Transmitted Infections

The recent pandemic has complicated the ability of doctors to diagnose and treat sexually transmitted infections. Many sexual health clinics that would normally screen patients shut down in the early stages of the pandemic, with approximately 80 percent of such clinics suspending services or shutting down completely. Additionally, routine healthcare was suspended as hospitals were – and in some cases remain – overwhelmed with coronavirus cases, further limiting testing and treatment. Contact tracers who previously kept track of sexually transmitted infections, such as chlamydia and gonorrhea, were greatly reduced in number and diverted to help with the pandemic efforts.

Concomitant with changes in tracing, most people's sexual appetites languished, as their energy seemed to be exhausted just trying to survive. Studies from around the world found that 40–60 percent of people reduced their number of sexual partners or the frequency of sex during the pandemic. As a consequence, we saw a substantial decline in the rates of sexually transmitted infections early on in the pandemic, although that has changed recently as social restrictions have eased. With the lifting of some restrictions, people who had previously limited casual sex during the pandemic have restarted their pre-pandemic behaviors.

Lessons from Historical Pandemics

If we look back to the bubonic plague of the thirteenth century, we see how pandemics can shape sexual life and it is not that uncommon compared to the current COVID-19 pandemic. In the thirteenth century, couples separated themselves in the home, and were not even allowed to talk.

There was similar misinformation about the plague with common social perceptions that immorality and illicit sexual relationships had caused the problem in the first place. Physicians advised physical distancing and abstinence from all forms of sexual intimacy, as sexual activity was considered to be a means by which the infection spread.

Just over 100 years ago, the "Spanish" flu pandemic occurred and seems to have affected our sex lives similarly to what we are seeing currently. During the Spanish flu of 1918, social distancing measures were used. The commonly quoted "You are your safest sexual partner" gained popularity. Some cities established kissing bans and protocols to curb the spread of the virus. There were some restrictions where people were told not to hug or kiss the soldiers returning from war because they might bring the virus with them. During the Spanish flu pandemic, people become more averse to sexual contact, and then, once the pandemic ended, there was a period in which people sought out extensive social and sexual interactions, a type of roaring 1920s response.

During the SARS (severe acute respiratory syndrome) outbreak of 2002–2004, research showed that there was an increase in sexual dysfunction, decreased arousal, and increased marital discord. Long-term psychosocial outcomes of healthcare workers dealing with SARS demonstrated an increase in erectile dysfunction, lack of sexual satisfaction in partners, and heightened performance anxiety. This in turn seemed to contribute to professional burnout, work stress, absenteeism, substance abuse, and depressive disorders. Similarly, in the case of COVID-19, healthcare workers who did not self-quarantine themselves to prevent interaction with their families reported problems with guilt and fear, which in turn affected interpersonal relationships, closeness, and sexual practices, and led to emotional distancing in couples. As was seen previously too, frontline healthcare workers have experienced disproportionate stress and reductions in their mental health and well-being during the COVID-19 pandemic.

Pandemics and Forced Abstinence

Sexual abstinence is when a person refrains from some or all aspects of sexual activity. In infectious disease outbreaks, abstinence is considered to be the safest practice to prevent spread. For decades, the psychological effects of sexual abstinence have been debated in all age groups. The traditional viewpoint has suggested that there may be beneficial effects of abstinence on self-control, spirituality, and well-being, but these are found in research where individuals practiced abstinence as a voluntary lifestyle. During infectious disease outbreaks, it is more of an "imposed abstinence" to prevent spread.

In contrast, sex is often considered to be a stress reliever and an indicator of well-being in couples, and forms an essential parameter of relationship dynamics. For sexually active couples, not being able to be intimate due to physical distancing or fear of infection can be traumatic and impact self-esteem and well-being. Many people can feel lonely in the absence of close contact with their partners. This becomes more concerning in couples who have just moved in together where sex has been seen as a way to emotionally bond and therefore increases the sense of emotional closeness among couples. Chronic sexual repression has been shown to affect performance anxiety and sexual confidence, which can eventually lead to arousal disorders, anorgasmia (inability to have orgasms), and erectile dysfunction. It can also increase the risk of chronic diseases such as diabetes, hypertension, and cardiovascular illness. Of course, psychological distress and sexual abstinence have been shown to have a bidirectional relationship, as increased stress can result in people avoiding sex. This factor becomes vital during disasters such as COVID-19 as the financial crisis, unemployment, fear of infection, health anxiety, travel restrictions, and uncertainty all contribute to the collective stress and hence changes in sexual behavior. Prolonged sexual abstinence might also lead to the emergence of high-risk sexual behavior, substance abuse, gambling, and compulsive self-gratification as harmful coping strategies.

Discussing Sexual Health during a Pandemic

Sexual health and well-being should be a priority discussion during this or other pandemics. For single people, technology, a form of digital intimacy, can play a vital role for both social and sexual connectedness. Allowing people to feel that technological intimacy is a legitimate form of sexual health during any forced quarantine may relieve the shame of the behavior and allow people the stress reduction that sexual expression often affords. Of course, emerging from a pandemic requires that we also further discuss how to be intimate again. As in the case of Brian, we may feel that we no longer have the social or sexual skills to meet someone and so need to be re-educated about healthy sexuality. Research has found that emerging from the pandemic, and re-adapting to life outside the home and to social contact, can be difficult for many people – and this will in turn be expected to impact the ability to re-establish dating and intimacy. The data show that difficulty adjusting to life "after lockdown" was linked to increases in mental health problems experienced during or prior to the pandemic.

Sexual health is part of our larger physical and mental health. Therefore, any discussion of healthy sexuality needs to address those issues that influence our sexuality, such as stress, poor self-esteem, financial problems, and relationship issues. In the case of Deidre, learning to address the relationship issues and her own stressors seems necessary for her overall sexual well-being. This can be accomplished in many ways including individual and couples therapy.

Summary

In this chapter, we have seen that the COVID-19 pandemic has affected people's sex lives in profoundly different ways, depending on context. For some, the pandemic has led to more social isolation or arguments with partners, frustration, and reductions in intimacy. For others, the pandemic has led to strengthening of partnership bonds and greater intimacy, or meeting new partners using technology in a creative way for the first time (stepping outside the usual "comfort zone" in a positive way). That being said, overall there has been a drop in sexual partners and sexually transmitted diseases, with an increase in the use of online pornography.

Some of the societal changes in sexual behaviors arising from the current pandemic are mirrored by what we know about previous pandemics, but at the same time, we did not have internet technology during previous pandemics: this is a crucial difference. Technology has pervaded our lives and both helped and hindered in radical ways. As we emerge from COVID-19 social restrictions and the aftermath, it seems likely that a sizable proportion of people will struggle to adapt to a "new normal" existence. While returning to "normal" may be a welcome relief to some in terms of sex, for others it will present major new difficulties.

APPENDIX: LIST OF RESOURCES

This section lists providers of information and support for sex and relationship issues. Often these resources can be helpful and relevant to people in other countries too.

Global

World Health Organization (WHO). Sexual Health. Provides educational information and fact sheets about key aspects of sex and public health (e.g. sexually transmitted infections, contraception, HIV/AIDs, and adolescent pregnancy): www.who.int/health-topics /sexual-health

World Health Organization (WHO). Sexuality Education. Advice and educational materials about sexuality education, relevant to educators: www.euro.who.int/en/health-topics/Life-stages/sexual-and-reproductive-health/areas-of-work/young-people/sexuality-education

USA

Centers for Disease Control and Prevention (CDC). Sexual Health. Offers information and links to other resources on many important topics: www.cdc.gov/sexualhealth/Default.html

Planned Parenthood. Includes a search tool to find clinics, and information about topics such as sexually transmitted infections and contraception: www.plannedparenthood.org/

UK

Mind. Provides support for a variety of mental health issues. Mind has branches in different parts of the country: www.mind.org.uk/

National Society for Prevention of Cruelty to Children (NSPCC). Offers advice and support for young people and adults (including parents in relation to their children). Has a telephone support line for young people, and for adults. Includes guidance on avoiding abusive relationships and risky situations: www.nspcc.org.uk/

Relate. Provides advice and counseling for couples: www.relate.org.uk/

Sexual Advice Association. Aims to improve the sexual health and wellbeing of men and women, and raise awareness of sexual conditions and problems and how to get support for them: https://sexualadviceassociation.co.uk/

Australia and New Zealand

Health Direct, Australia. Sexual Health. Advice about safe sex, contraception, sexually transmitted infections, sexual problems, and pregnancy. Includes a symptom checker tool for sexual health and look-up facilities for clinical services: www.healthdirect.gov.au/sexual-health

Health Navigator, New Zealand. Sexual Health for Young People. Provides top tips and links to many sources of support for young people: www.healthnavigator.org.nz/healthy-living/s/sexual-health-help-for-young-people/

Ministry of Health, New Zealand. Information on many aspects of sexual health along with links to key resources for the public and professionals. www.health.govt.nz/our-work/preventative-health-wellness/sexual-and-reproductive-health

New Zealand Sexual Health Society. Guidelines and education about a large variety of topics and for specific populations and minority groups. Also has a list of clinics: www.nzshs.org/

Raisingchildren.net.au. Links for key sexual health advice and support services for younger people in Australia. https://raisingchildren

.net.au/grown-ups/services-support/services-families-of-teens
/teens-sexual-health

Sexual Health and Family Planning Australia. Various educational materials about sex and sexual health, as well as a tool to find a local sexual health clinic: http://shfpa.org.au/

South Africa

Southern African Sexual Health Association. Dedicated to the provision and promotion of sexual health within the healthcare professions, and the development and advancement of sexual therapy, counseling, and education: https://sasha.org.za/

SELECTED LITERATURE
AND FURTHER READING

Chapter 1: Introduction

Beckmeyer JJ, Herbenick D, Fu TC, Dodge B, Fortenberry JD. Pleasure during adolescents' most recent partnered sexual experience: findings from a U.S. probability survey. *Arch Sex Behav* 2021;**50**(6):2423–34. doi:10.1007/s10508-021-02026-4

Derbyshire KL, Grant JE. Compulsive sexual behavior: a review of the literature. *J Behav Addict* 2015;4(2):37–43. doi:10.1556/2006.4.2015.003

Longmore MA, Eng AL, Giordano PC, Manning WD. Parenting and adolescents' sexual initiation. *J Marriage Fam* 2009;71(4): 969–82. doi:10.1111/j.1741-3737.2009.00647.x

Madkour AS, de Looze M, Ma P, et al. Macro-level age norms for the timing of sexual initiation and adolescents' early sexual initiation in 17 European countries. *J Adolesc Health* 2014;**55**(1): 114–21. doi:10.1016/j.jadohealth.2013.12.008

Magnusson BM, Crandall A, Evans K. Early sexual debut and risky sex in young adults: the role of low self-control. *BMC Public Health* 2019;**19**(1):1483. doi:10.1186/s12889-019-7734-9

Chapter 2: Sex and Desire

Boly M, Coleman MR, Davis MH, et al. When thoughts become action: an fMRI paradigm to study volitional brain activity in non-communicative brain injured patients. *Neuroimage* 2007;**36**(3):979–92. doi:10.1016/j.neuroimage.2007.02.047

Crusius J, Mussweiler T. When people want what others have: the impulsive side of envious desire. *Emotion* 2012;**12**(1):142–53. doi:10.1037/a0023523

Dawson SJ, Suschinsky KD, Lalumière ML. Habituation of sexual responses in men and women: a test of the preparation hypothesis of women's genital responses. *J Sex Med* 2013;**10**(4): 990–1000. doi:10.1111/jsm.12032

Filgueiras A, Quintas Conde EF, Hall CR. The neural basis of kinesthetic and visual imagery in sports: an ALE meta – analysis. *Brain Imaging Behav* 2018;**12**(5), 1513–23. doi:10.1007/s11682-017-9813-9

Higgins JA, Trussell J, Moore NB, Davidson JK. Virginity lost, satisfaction gained? Physiological and psychological sexual satisfaction at heterosexual debut. *J Sex Res* 2010;**47**(4):384–94. doi:10.1080/00224491003774792

Joyal CC, Cossette A, Lapierre V. What exactly is an unusual sexual fantasy? *J Sex Med* 2015;**12**(2):328–40. doi:10.1111/jsm.12734

Voon V, Mole TB, Banca P, et al. Neural correlates of sexual cue reactivity in individuals with and without compulsive sexual behaviours. *PLoS One* 2014;**9**(7):e102419. doi:10.1371/journal.pone.0102419

Chapter 3:   Development Issues around Sex

Aron AR, Robbins TW, Poldrack RA. Inhibition and the right inferior frontal cortex: one decade on. *Trends Cogn Sci* 2014;**18**(4):177–85. doi:10.1016/j.tics.2013.12.003

Bersamin M, Todd M, Fisher DA, et al. Parenting practices and adolescent sexual behavior: a longitudinal study. *J Marriage Fam* 2008;**70**(1):97–112. doi:10.1111/j.1741-3737.2007.00464.x

Djalovski A, Kinreich S, Zagoory-Sharon O, Feldman R. Social dialogue triggers biobehavioral synchrony of partners' endocrine response via sex-specific, hormone-specific, attachment-specific mechanisms. *Sci Rep* 2021;**11**(1):12421. doi:10.1038/s41598-021-91626-0

Heywood W, Patrick K, Smith AM, Pitts MK. Associations between early first sexual intercourse and later sexual and reproductive outcomes: a systematic review of population-based data. *Arch Sex Behav* 2015;**44**(3):531–69. doi:10.1007/s10508-014-0374-3

Kendler KS, Thornton LM, Gilman SE, Kessler RC. Sexual orientation in a U.S. national sample of twin and nontwin sibling pairs. *Am J Psychiatry* 2000;**157**(11):1843–46. doi:10.1176/appi.ajp.157.11.1843

Meeus W, Vollebergh W, Branje S, et al. On imbalance of impulse control and sensation seeking and adolescent risk: an intra-individual developmental test of the dual systems and maturational imbalance models. *J Youth Adolesc* 2021;**50**(5): 827–40. doi:10.1007/s10964-021-01419-x

Palmer MJ, Clarke L, Ploubidis GB, et al. Prevalence and correlates of 'sexual competence' at first heterosexual intercourse among young people in Britain. *BMJ Sex Reprod Health* 2019;**45**:127–37. doi:10.1136/bmjsrh-2018-200160

Peper JS, Dahl RE. Surging hormones: brain–behavior interactions during puberty. *Curr Dir Psychol Sci* 2013;**22**(2):134–9. doi:10.1177/0963721412473755

Petersen JL, Hyde JS. Gender differences in sexual attitudes and behaviors: a review of meta-analytic results and large datasets. *J Sex Res* 2011; **48** (2–3):149–65. doi:10.1080/00224499.2011.551851

Robbins CL, Schick V, Reece M, et al. Prevalence, frequency, and associations of masturbation with partnered sexual behaviors among US adolescents. *Arch Pediatr Adolesc Med* 2011;**165**(12): 1087–93. doi:10.1001/archpediatrics.2011.142

Volkow ND, Michaelides M, Baler R. The neuroscience of drug reward and addiction. *Physiol Rev* 2019;**99**(4):2115–40. doi: 10.1152/physrev.00014.2018

Wang KS, Smith DV, Delgado MR. Using fMRI to study reward processing in humans: past, present, and future. *J Neurophysiol* 2016;**115**(3):1664–78. doi:10.1152/jn.00333.2015

Chapter 4:   Healthy Sex

Blanchflower DG. Is happiness U-shaped everywhere? Age and subjective well-being in 145 countries. *J Popul Econ* 2020;**34**(2): 575–624. doi: 10.1007/s00148-020-00797-z

Fileborn B, Thorpe R, Hawkes G, et al. Sex, desire and pleasure: considering the experiences of older Australian women. *Sex Relation Ther* 2015;**30**(1):117–30. doi:10.1080/14681994.2014.936722

Fisher TD, Moore ZT, Pittenger MJ. Sex on the brain?: an examination of frequency of sexual cognitions as a function of gender, erotophilia, and social desirability. *J Sex Res* 2012;**49**(1): 69–77. doi:10.1080/00224499.2011.565429

Giles GG, Severi G, English DR, et al. Sexual factors and prostate cancer. *BJU Int* 2003;**92**(3):211–16. doi:10.1046/j.1464-410X.2003.04319.x

Hald GM. Gender differences in pornography consumption among young heterosexual Danish adults. *Arch Sex Behav* 2006;**35**(5): 577–85. doi:10.1007/s10508-006-9064-0. PMID: 17039402

Hurlbert DF, Whittaker KE. The role of masturbation in marital and sexual satisfaction: a comparative study of female masturbators and nonmasturbators. *J Sex Educ Ther* 1991;**17**(4): 272–82. doi:10.1080/01614576.1991.11074029

Michalek AM, Mettlin C, Priore RL. Prostate cancer mortality among Catholic priests. *J Surg Oncol* 1981;**17**(2):129–33. doi:10.1002/jso.2930170205

Rider JR, Wilson KM, Sinnott JA, et al. Ejaculation frequency and risk of prostate cancer: updated results with an additional decade of follow-up. *Eur Urol* 2016;**70**(6):974–82. doi:10.1016/j.eururo.2016.03.027

Ross RK, Deapen DM, Casagrande JT, Paganini-Hill A, Henderson BE. A cohort study of mortality from cancer of the prostate in Catholic priests. *Br J Cancer* 1981;**43**(2):233–5. doi:10.1038/bjc.1981.34

Waldinger MD, Quinn P, Dilleen M, et al. A multinational population survey of intravaginal ejaculation latency time. *J Sex Med* 2005;**2**(4):492–7. doi: 10.1111/j.1743-6109.2005.00070.x

Chapter 5: Too Little Sex

Bancroft J. The endocrinology of sexual arousal. *J Endocrinol* 2005;**186**(3):411–27. doi:10.1677/joe.1.06233

Ben Zion IZ, Tessler R, Cohen L, et al. Polymorphisms in the dopamine D4 receptor gene (*DRD4*) contribute to individual differences in human sexual behavior: desire, arousal and sexual function. *Mol Psychiatry* 2006;**11**(8):782–6. doi:10.1038/sj.mp.4001832

Burger HG, Papalia MA. A clinical update on female androgen insufficiency – testosterone testing and treatment in women presenting with low sexual desire. *Sex Health* 2006;**3**(2):73–8. doi:10.1071/sh05055

Hardman RK, Gardner DJ. Sexual anorexia: a look at inhibited sexual desire. *J Sex Educ Thera* 1986;**12**:1, 55–9. doi:10.1080/01614576.1986.11074863

Liu L, Kang R, Zhao S, et al. Sexual dysfunction in patients with obstructive sleep apnea: a systematic review and meta-analysis. *J Sex Med* 2015;**12**(10):1992–2003. doi:10.1111/jsm.12983

Nappi RE, Terreno E, Martini E, et al. Hypoactive sexual desire disorder: can we treat it with drugs? *Sexual and Relationship Therapy*, 2010;25(3), 264–74, doi:10.1080/14681991003669030

Quinn-Nilas C, Benson L, Milhausen RR, Buchholz AC, Goncalves M. The relationship between body image and domains of sexual functioning among heterosexual, emerging adult women. *Sex Med* 2016;4(3):e182–9. doi:10.1016/j.esxm.2016.02.004

Chapter 6: Too Much Sex

Chatzittofis A, Boström AE, Öberg KG, et al. Normal testosterone but higher luteinizing hormone plasma levels in men with hypersexual disorder. *Sex Med* 2020;8(2):243–50. doi:10.1016/j.esxm.2020.02.005

Derbyshire KL, Grant JE. Neurocognitive findings in compulsive sexual behavior: a preliminary study. *J Behav Addict* 2015;4(2):35–6. doi:10.1556/2006.4.2015.004

Derbyshire KL, Grant JE. Compulsive sexual behavior: a review of the literature. *J Behav Addict* 2015;4(2):37–43. doi:10.1556/2006.4.2015.003

Kaplan MS, Krueger RB. Diagnosis, assessment, and treatment of hypersexuality. *J Sex Res* 2010;47(2):181–98. doi:10.1080/00224491003592863

Kowalewska E, Gola M, Kraus SW, Lew-Starowicz M. Spotlight on compulsive sexual behavior disorder: a systematic review of research on women. *Neuropsychiatr Dis Treat* 2020;16:2025–43. doi:10.2147/NDT.S221540

Kraus SW, Krueger RB, Briken P, et al. Compulsive sexual behaviour disorder in the ICD-11. *World Psychiatry* 2018;17(1):109–10. doi:10.1002/wps.20499

Kuzma JM, Black DW. Epidemiology, prevalence, and natural history of compulsive sexual behavior. *Psychiatr Clin North Am* 2008;**31**(4):603–11. doi:10.1016/j.psc.2008.06.005

Odlaug BL, Lust K, Schreiber LR, et al. Compulsive sexual behavior in young adults. *Ann Clin Psychiatry* 2013;**25**(3):193–200.

Slavin MN, Scoglio AAJ, Blycker GR, Potenza MN, Kraus SW. Child sexual abuse and compulsive sexual behavior: a systematic literature review. *Curr Addict Rep* 2020;**7**(1):76–88. doi:10.1007/s40429-020-00298-9

Chapter 7:   Sex and Physical Health

Chou KL, Ng ISF, Yu KM. Lifetime abstention of sexual intercourse and health in middle-aged and older adults: results from wave 2 of the National Epidemiologic Survey on Alcohol and Related Conditions. *Arch Sex Behav* 2014;**43**:891–900. doi:10.1007/s10508-013-0176-z

Ebrahim S, May M, Ben Shlomo Y, et al. Sexual intercourse and risk of ischaemic stroke and coronary heart disease: the Caerphilly study. *J Epidemiol Community Health* 2002;**56**(2): 99–102. doi:10.1136/jech.56.2.99

Hambach A, Evers S, Summ O, Husstedt IW, Frese A. The impact of sexual activity on idiopathic headaches: an observational study. *Cephalalgia* 2013;**33**(6):384–9. doi:10.1177/0333102413476374

Kouidrat Y, Pizzol D, Cosco T, et al. High prevalence of erectile dysfunction in diabetes: a systematic review and meta-analysis of 145 studies. *Diabet Med* 2017;**34**(9):1185–92. doi:10.1111/dme.13403

Momenimovahed Z, Salehiniya H. Epidemiological characteristics of and risk factors for breast cancer in the world. *Breast Cancer (Dove Med Press)*. 2019;**11**:151–64. doi:10.2147/BCTT.S176070

Nemec ED, Mansfield L, Kennedy JW. Heart rate and blood pressure responses during sexual activity in normal males. *Am Heart J* 1976;**92**(3):274–7. doi:10.1016/s0002-8703(76)80106-8

Palmeri ST, Kostis JB, Casazza L, et al. Heart rate and blood pressure response in adult men and women during exercise and sexual activity. *Am J Cardiol* 2007;**100**(12):1795–801. doi:10.1016/j.amjcard.2007.07.040

Whipple B, Komisaruk BR. Elevation of pain threshold by vaginal stimulation in women. *Pain* 1985;**21**(4):357–67. doi:10.1016/0304-3959(85)90164-2

Wright H, Jenks RA. Sex on the brain! Associations between sexual activity and cognitive function in older age. *Age Ageing* 2016;**45**(2):313–17, doi:10.1093/ageing/afv197

Chapter 8: Drinking, Drugs, and Sex

Chou NH, Huang YJ, Jiann BP. The impact of illicit use of amphetamine on male sexual functions. *J Sex Med* 2015;**12**(8): 1694–702. doi:10.1111/jsm.12926

Fillmore MT. Acute alcohol-induced impairment of cognitive functions: past and present findings. *Int J Disabil Hum Dev* 2007;**6**(2):115–26. doi:10.1515/IJDHD.2007.6.2.115

Fonseca BM, Rebelo I. Cannabis and cannabinoids in reproduction and fertility: where we stand. *Reprod Sci* 2021 (Epub ahead of print). doi:10.1007/s43032-021-00588-1

George WH. Alcohol and sexual health behavior: "What we know and how we know it". *J Sex Res* 2019;**56**(4–5):409–24. doi:10.1080/00224499.2019.1588213

Lawn W, Aldridge A, Xia R, Winstock AR. Substance-linked sex in heterosexual, homosexual, and bisexual men and women: an online, cross-sectional "global drug survey"

report. *J Sex Med* 2019;**16**(5):721–32. doi:10.1016/
j.jsxm.2019.02.018

Lynn B, Gee A, Zhang L, Pfaus JG. Effects of cannabinoids on
female sexual function. *Sex Med Rev* 2020;**8**(1):18–27.
doi:10.1016/j.sxmr.2019.07.004

Parrott AC. MDMA in humans: factors which affect the
neuropsychobiological profiles of recreational ecstasy users, the
integrative role of bioenergetic stress. *J Psychopharmacol*
2006;**20**(2):147–63. doi:10.1177/0269881106063268

Pizzol D, Demurtas J, Stubbs B, et al. Relationship between
cannabis use and erectile dysfunction: a systematic review and
meta-analysis. *Am J Mens Health* 2019;**13**(6):1557988319892464.
doi:10.1177/1557988319892464

Sivaratnam L, Selimin DS, Abd Ghani SR, Nawi HM, Nawi AM.
Behavior-related erectile dysfunction: a systematic review and
meta-analysis. *J Sex Med* 2021;**18**(1):121–43. doi:10.1016/
j.jsxm.2020.09.009

Chapter 10:   Sex and Digital Technology

Bőthe B, Tóth-Király I, Potenza MN, Orosz G, Demetrovics Z.
High-frequency pornography use may not always be
problematic. *J Sex Med* 2020;**17**(4):793–811. doi:10.1016/
j.jsxm.2020.01.007

Bőthe B, Tóth-Király I, Bella N, et al. Why do people watch
pornography? The motivational basis of pornography use.
Psychol Addict Behav 2021;**35**(2):172–86. doi:10.1037/adb0000603

Bőthe B, Vaillancourt-Morel MP, Bergeron S. Associations
between pornography use frequency, pornography use
motivations, and sexual wellbeing in couples. *J Sex Res* 2021;
59(4):457–471. doi:10.1080/00224499.2021.1893261

Castro Á, Barrada JR. Dating apps and their sociodemographic
and psychosocial correlates: a systematic review.

Int J Environ Res Public Health 2020;17(18):6500. doi:10.3390/ijerph17186500

Choi EPH, Wong JYH, Lo HHM, et al. The impacts of using smartphone dating applications on sexual risk behaviours in college students in Hong Kong. *PLoS One* 2016;11(11):e0165394. doi:10.1371/journal.pone.0165394

Fineberg NA, Demetrovics Z, Stein DJ, et al. Manifesto for a European research network into Problematic Usage of the Internet. *Eur Neuropsychopharmacol* 2018;28(11):1232–46. doi:10.1016/j.euroneuro.2018.08.004

Fuss J, Bothe B. Cybersex (including sex robots). In: Stein DJ, Fineberg NA, Chamberlain SR, eds. *Mental Health In A Digital World*. Global Mental Health in Practice Series. London: Academic Press, 2022; 307–44.

Holtzhausen, N., Fitzgerald, K., Thakur, I. et al. Swipe-based dating applications use and its association with mental health outcomes: a cross-sectional study. *BMC Psychol* 2020;8(1):22. doi:10.1186/s40359-020-0373-1

Internet and Me. *Learning to Deal with Problematic Usage of the Internet*. COST Action on Problematic Usage of the Internet. Available from: www.internetandme.eu

Ioannidis K, Treder MS, Chamberlain SR, et al. Problematic internet use as an age-related multifaceted problem: evidence from a two-site survey. *Addict Behav* 2018;81:157–66. doi:10.1016/j.addbeh.2018.02.017

Lewczuk K, Wójcik A, Gola, M. Increase in the prevalence of online pornography use: objective data analysis from the period between 2004 and 2016 in Poland. *Arch Sex Behav* 2022;51(2):1157–71. doi:10.1007/s10508-021-02090-w

Park BY, Wilson G, Berger J, et al. Is internet pornography causing sexual dysfunctions? *Behav Sci (Basel)* 2018;8(6):17. doi:10.3390/bs6030017

Rochat L, Bianchi-Demicheli F, Aboujaoude E, Khazaal Y. The psychology of "swiping": a cluster analysis of the mobile dating app Tinder. *J Behav Addict* 2019;8(4):804–13. doi:10.1556/2006.8.2019.58

Vaillancourt-Morel MP, Rosen NO, Štulhofer A, Bosisio M, Bergeron S. Pornography use and sexual health among same-sex and mixed-sex couples: an event-level dyadic analysis. *Arch Sex Behav* 2021;50(2):667–81. doi: 10.1007/s10508-020-01839-z

Voon V, Mole TB, Banca P, et al. Neural correlates of sexual cue reactivity in individuals with and without compulsive sexual behaviours. *PLoS One* 2014;9(7):e102419. doi:10.1371/journal.pone.0102419

Chapter 11:   Diverse Aspects of Sex

Copen CE, Chandra A, Febo-Vazquez I. *Sexual Behavior, Sexual Attraction, and Sexual Orientation among Adults Aged 18–44 in the United States: Data from the 2011–2013 National Survey of Family Growth.* National Health Statistics Reports, No. 88. Hyattsville, MD, National Center for Health Statistics, 2016.

Davis DL, Whitten RG. The cross-cultural study of human sexuality. *Ann Rev Anthropol* 1987;16(1):69–98. doi:10.1146/annurev.an.16.100187.000441

Diamond LM. Sexual fluidity in male and females. *Curr Sex Health Rep* 2016;8:249–56. doi:10.1007/s11930-016-0092-z

Hines M. Prenatal endocrine influences on sexual orientation and on sexually differentiated childhood behavior. *Front Neuroendocrinol* 2011;32(2):170–82. doi:10.1016/j.yfrne.2011.02.006

King M, Semlyen J, Tai SS, et al. A systematic review of mental disorder, suicide, and deliberate self harm in lesbian, gay and bisexual people. *BMC Psychiatry* 2008;8:70. doi:10.1186/1471-244X-8-70

Luo L, Deng T, Zhao S, et al. Association between HIV infection and prevalence of erectile dysfunction: a systematic review and meta-analysis. *J Sex Med* 2017;14(9):1125–32. doi:10.1016/j.jsxm.2017.07.001

Sell RL, Wells JA, Wypij D. The prevalence of homosexual behavior and attraction in the United States, the United Kingdom and France: results of national population-based samples. *Arch Sex Behav* 1995;24(3):235–48. doi:10.1007/BF01541598

Chapter 12:   Sex and Pandemics

Ates E, Kazici HG, Yildiz AE, et al. Male sexual functions and behaviors in the age of COVID-19: evaluation of mid-term effects with online cross-sectional survey study. *Arch Ital Urol Androl* 2021;93(3):341–7. doi:10.4081/aiua.2021.3.341

Fineberg NA, Pellegrini L, Wellsted D, et al. Facing the "new normal": how adjusting to the easing of COVID-19 lockdown restrictions exposes mental health inequalities. *J Psychiatr Res* 2021;141:276–86. doi:10.1016/j.jpsychires.2021.07.001

Hampshire A, Hellyer PJ, Soreq E, et al. Associations between dimensions of behaviour, personality traits, and mental-health during the COVID-19 pandemic in the United Kingdom. *Nat Commun* 2021;12(1):4111. doi:10.1038/s41467-021-24365-5. (Erratum: *Nat Commun* 2021;12(1):5047.)

Hampshire A, Hellyer PJ, Trender W, Chamberlain SR. Insights into the impact on daily life of the COVID-19 pandemic and effective coping strategies from free-text analysis of people's collective experiences. *Interface Focus* 2021;11(6):20210051. doi:10.1098/rsfs.2021.0051

Lau WK, Ngan LH, Chan RC, Wu WK, Lau BW. Impact of COVID-19 on pornography use: evidence from big data analyses. *PLoS One* 2021;**16**(12):e0260386. doi:10.1371/journal.pone.0260386

Mukherjee TI, Khan AG, Dasgupta A, Samari G. Reproductive justice in the time of COVID-19: a systematic review of the indirect impacts of COVID-19 on sexual and reproductive health. *Reprod Health* 2021;**18**(1):252. doi:10.1186/s12978-021-01286-6

Saarentausta K, Ivarsson L, Jacobsson S, et al. Potential impact of the COVID-19 pandemic on the national and regional incidence, epidemiology and diagnostic testing of chlamydia and gonorrhoea in Sweden, 2020. *APMIS* 2022;**130**(1):34–42. doi:10.1111/apm.13191

Tarin-Vicente EJ, Sendagorta Cudos E, Servera Negre G, et al. Sexually transmitted infections during the first wave of the COVID-19 pandemic in Spain. *Actas Dermosifiliogr* 2021 (Epub ahead of print). doi:10.1016/j.adengl.2021.11.024

INDEX